YO-DRX-053

5119

Neff

World University Library

The World University Library is an international series
of books, each of which has been specially commissioned.
The authors are leading scientists and scholars from all over
the world who, in an age of increasing specialization, see the
need for a broad, up-to-date presentation of their subject.
The aim is to provide authoritative introductory books for
students which will be of interest also to the general
reader. Publication of the series takes place in Britain,
France, Germany, Holland, Italy, Spain, Sweden and
the United States.

Magnus Pyke

Man and Food

World University Library

McGraw-Hill Book Company
New York Toronto

© Magnus Pyke 1970
All rights reserved. No part of this publication may be reproduced,
stored in a retrieval system, or transmitted, in any form or by any
means electronic, mechanical, photocopying, recording or
otherwise, without the prior permission of the Copyright owner.

Phototypeset by BAS Printers Limited, Wallop, Hampshire, England
Manufactured by LIBREX, Italy

Contents

1 Scientific need and human choice

The modern understanding of food science can be said to have started with the penetrating observation of Antoine Lavoisier at the end of the eighteenth century that 'la vie est une fonction chimique' – life is a chemical process. Once this idea had been accepted, and the contrary notion that life was a mysterious force the nature of which was inexplicable by rational methods of investigation was abandoned, progress became possible in understanding the composition of foods and their function in maintaining the vigour, growth and health of the human body. First came the elucidation of the fuel-value of foods. This was done by Lavoisier himself with great insight and with a degree of accuracy that has stood up to two hundred years of scrutiny. He measured it in terms of 'pouces'; today it is done in terms of kilocalories, each defined as the amount of heat energy needed to raise the temperature of a litre of water one degree centigrade. Next the main chemical components of food were distinguished. Fat was seen to be palpably different in composition from the so-called carbohydrates, the sugars and starches. Both of these are, in turn, different from protein, of which lean meat, egg, cheese and the gluten of flour are mainly composed.

These, the main substances of food, are all organic and as such their molecular structure is made up of a complex framework of carbon atoms. It only required simple chemical manipulation to distinguish these from the inorganic components, calcium, magnesium, iron, etc. Before the nineteenth century was over, a formidable body of knowledge had accrued and there were grounds for the confidence expressed by certain Victorian savants that the scientific understanding of food chemistry was complete. We now know that the existence of a group of diverse organic substances, present in food only in amounts of a few parts per million, yet of capital nutritional importance, was just about to be unfolded. These were the vitamins. But although in the present century nutritional science has evolved to a remarkable degree, as is described in chapter six, we should deceive ourselves if we too overlooked the extent of our current ignorance.

To know that life is a chemical process is at least to understand the nature of the problem which has to be solved but it does not imply that the problem is solved. Today, although we know more about food chemistry than our nineteenth-century grandparents, there is even yet much more to be known. The commodities that are used for food are themselves living things. It follows, therefore, that food analysis is not a simple matter of chemistry but itself comprises something of the complexity of life chemistry. For example, meat is in the main the muscular tissue of the animal from which it is derived. Muscle is mostly protein. But 'protein' is the name not of a single compound but of a group, each member of which has a different chemical composition. And mingled with the protein are various other compounds which, when the meat animal was alive, made its muscle into an active, self-renewing biological machine. There are breakdown products of protein, compounds of protein and carbohydrate, so-called 'extractives' which, in chemical terms, are *purines* and *pyrimidines*, but which, in culinary terms, contribute to the 'meaty' flavour of a joint of meat. Besides these there are connective tissue (which is 'gristle') and interstitial fat.

The more deeply food science is studied the more complex – and the more interesting – it becomes. To keep his milk free from contamination, a prudent modern farmer will spray his cowshed with DDT to suppress flies. The cows absorb a trace of DDT themselves and excrete it in their milk. The children who drink the milk, and the calves which are raised on it, also absorb DDT into their tissues, where it can be detected by chemical analysis. DDT is an artificial substance; there are, however, a variety of natural substances that may be stored in animal tissues. Liver, for example, besides its other functions in the animal from which it comes, is also a storage organ. The concentration of iron in liver is high; it also serves as a store of vitamin A and for several of the B-vitamins. Because of its ability to store such compounds and, by storing them provide a concentrated source of them when it is eaten as a food, liver is accepted as a nutritious foodstuff. This, however, may not be so for the livers of all species of animals or for all circumstances. Eskimos were aware, before the days of science, that the liver of polar bears was poisonous. Scientific investigations showed that the toxic agent in it was the enormously high concentration of vitamin A, which the bears acquire from eating large amounts of fish which themselves have quantities of vitamin A in their liver oils.

Fish, like meat, is mainly composed of protein, but here again it must be recognised that there are a large number of other components, some present in quite large proportions, some in trace amounts and others, it can confidently be predicted, not yet discovered. The fat content of such fish as herring varies depending on the physiological state of the fish. After fish have been caught a series of chemical changes begin to occur. This is obvious from the change in appearance and taste as the fish begin to age and become stale. Then again, not all species of fish possess the same biochemical systems for coping with the problems of living. Dogfish and sharks deal with the business of survival in salt water in a way that is different from that followed by other fish and thus produces certain chemical changes in the composition of their flesh.

Cereals, of which wheat is the most important in Western countries and rice in the East, are sometimes thought to be merely sources of 'starch'. In fact, their composition is remarkably complex. They contain protein, varying proportions of fat, and significant amounts of the group of vitamins commonly called the 'vitamin B complex'. The amounts of all these components and the distribution of each in the various structures of which the cereals are made up has an important bearing on the chemical composition and on the consequent nutritional value of the commodities made from them. And besides the significance of the amount of each separate component, the relative amounts of two or more may have a bearing on the food value of a particular cereal. For example, the disease pellagra was recognised to occur most commonly among populations using maize as their staple cereal. This disease occurs when insufficient of the vitamin niacin is available. Yet the amount of niacin present in maize was not found to be significantly less than in other cereals. It was later discovered that the protein of maize was of a chemical composition which differed in one significant respect from protein in wheat or rice and that it was the interaction of the content of both niacin and of the maize protein which together led to nutritional deficiency causing pellagra.

Understanding of the chemistry of fruit and vegetables has gone through a number of phases and illustrates very strikingly the way in which food science has developed. At first, when interest was concentrated on the principal food components – protein, carbohydrate and fat – it was thought that fruit and vegetables, which are mostly water, made a negligible contribution to the diet. Later, however, when it was discovered that they contained vitamin C, they were esteemed almost solely for this and little attention was paid to the composition of the remainder of their dry substance. It is only now that the chemical components of cabbage, potatoes, onion and the like are being studied in detail. Firstly, the protein of green vegetables, although it is not present in very large amount, may make a useful contribution to the diet. On the other hand, new knowledge is coming to light showing that there are substances which, although present in quite small proportions, may affect health. Cabbage, for example, possesses a component which influences goitre, onions contain a substance affecting anaemia, and potatoes contain a substance, solanin, which under certain circumstances may exert a harmful effect on people consuming the vegetable. The lesson to be learned is that although the body of food chemistry that has already been established is large, there is much more still to know.

But while life is, as has been truly said, a chemical process, an understanding of the chemical compounds by which it is maintained is only part of food science. People must eat what they need, to be sure, but in real life they choose what they like. Health will be maintained, therefore, only when they like what they need. A major purpose of the processes by which foods are prepared for consumption, whether this be by cooking or by the most up-to-date methods of food technology, is to make food palatable.

It is sometimes believed that the main effect of cooking is to damage or destroy the nutritional value of the cooked food. This is not so; not only does cooking make food more agreeable to eat, it also makes it in many respects more nourishing. The main component of flour is starch. The starch molecules are composed of long chains of carbon atoms which, as the grain of wheat gradually ripens on the ear, become tightly wound, rather like a ball of wool, and take the form of granules. When starch is cooked in the baking of bread or the boiling of potatoes, the starch granules burst in the heat and their contents are very much more readily digested and absorbed. If the heating is carried further, as in the toasting of bread or the browning of potatoes in a pan, the starch molecules themselves are partly split into *dextrins* which contribute to the pleasant digestible character of toast and fried potatoes.

The molecular configuration of the complex molecules of protein is similarly changed by the heat of cooking when meat is roasted. The meat contracts and, as with starch molecules, the molecule of protein may also be partly degraded when the conditions of cooking become more extreme. When this occurs one of the effects is often to make the food component more readily available to the body. But parallel with the simple splitting of the large molecules of protein or starch, other and more complex chemical reactions take place leading to the formation of a variety of compounds which are responsible for the taste and smell of cooked foods. It is only within the last few years that sufficiently sensitive analytical methods have become available to enable these substances to be identified. The results of numerous researches show that the flavours and aromas which render cooked foods attractive and which, by doing so, contribute both to human nutrition and to human satisfaction, are derived from a complex mixture of substances, some of which are present in only minute concentrations.

To study food in relation to human wellbeing to any degree of comprehensiveness, it is necessary to deal with three interlocking areas of knowledge. The first of these is the chemical composition of different food commodities and the amount of the different nutrients of which foods are composed which are required for physiological wellbeing. The first few chapters of this book deal with these matters. Next there is the question of what people like and what they choose to eat. In this context, one must consider what constitutes 'good quality' in a food and how foods can be processed and converted into articles which consumers will be eager to buy. But the third topic is as important as the other two. People do not exist in a vacuum, neither do they separate the satisfaction of their requirement for food from the diverse other competing requirements which must also be satisfied.

A modern community is a complex biological organism. Nutritional deficiency, even starvation, is primarily due to lack of food or lack of the right food but the immediate cause may be something quite different, shortage of money, perhaps, or religious taboo inhibiting people from eating food of a particular sort even if it is available. Some of these things are touched on in the later chapters of this book. There is one further important cause of malnutrition and ill-health; this is ignorance. Ignorance of food chemistry can be dispelled or at least reduced to the limit of our present-day understanding. Ignorance of food technology can also be overcome. Perhaps ignorance of how populations behave and the factors that make them do so is most difficult to overcome because, if the behaviour of the peoples of the world, and their inability to bring food surpluses in one country to hungry people in another is any indication, the wisdom to overcome it is not yet available.

Part 1

Commodities selected as food

2 Meat and fish

Meat

It is important to remember that the composition of meat and its value as food depend on the animal producing it. One of the most significant factors is the age of the animal. For example, when a lamb is born, it is all head, shins and shanks, which are parts of low food value. As the lamb grows, first of all its body lengthens and then it thickens. This means that the proportion of head and shanks becomes less. A wave of growth, as it were, starts at the head and moves backwards while, simultaneously, lesser waves start at the feet and tail and move forwards. All these waves meet at the loin which is the most valuable part of the animal as meat. If one considers these developments in terms of the components of which they are made up, it may be said that bone is the earliest component to develop, muscle – that is lean meat – follows next, while last of all comes fat.

The effect of age is most strikingly seen when one considers what happens in quantitative terms. An animal shaped like a new born lamb provides only 53 lb of carcase meat for each 100 lb of live weight. But later on, the beast that has grown to the shape of an adult ram yields 67 lb of carcase meat for every 100 lb of live weight. There is, in fact, 17 per cent of bone in a new born lamb compared with only 4 per cent of bone in a ram.

There are two other factors in an animal which affect its effectiveness as a producer of meat. The first is the way it is fed. If it is well fed while it is young, the age changes in form and consequently in the composition of the carcase are accelerated. This means that the useful loin and the proportion of useful meat and fat on it develop more quickly. On the other hand, if the animal is given only a sparse ration, its head and bones, which have the first calls on the nutrients it consumes, will grow and the later maturing and more valuable parts will go short. The result will be a leggy beast with a big head which will provide comparatively little meat, and of poor quality. It is, therefore, an economical procedure for a stockfeeder who intends to produce animals for meat to ensure that they are

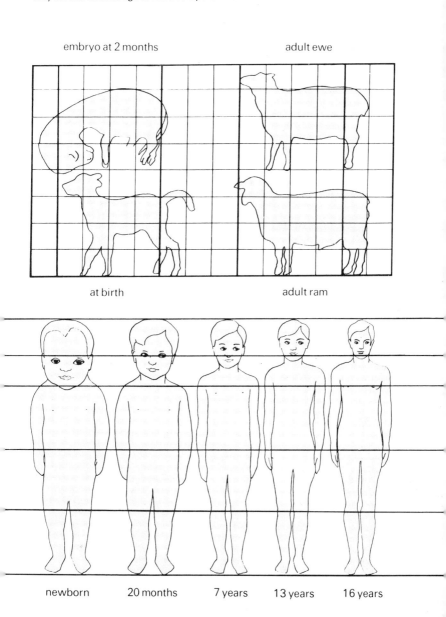

2·1 Different parts of animals' bodies grow at different rates, whether they are cattle or human beings. Consequently, if one is going to use them for meat, there will be different proportions of meat, fat and bone, depending on how they are fed and the age at which they are killed.

embryo at 2 months

adult ewe

at birth

adult ram

newborn   20 months   7 years   13 years   16 years

adequately fed during their growing period. Besides the effect of feeding the livestock on the amount and quality of the meat produced, the breeding of the beast is also important. So-called 'improved' breeds of animals respond much more to the effect of proper feeding. A pure-bred pig will yield more edible meat for each pound of feed it receives than a wild boar. The fundamental nature of these changes in body proportions is shown in figure 2·1 where the proportions of head and legs are shown for sheep and, as a matter of comparison, for man side by side. Although these changes are basic to the growth of the species, their timing and the precise extent to which they occur are, as has already been pointed out, affected by the nutritional history of the growing animal.

The relationship of fat to meat quality The meat from different parts of an animal differs in its composition. In a characteristic sheep bred for mutton the desirable meat from the loin is made up of 36 per cent of fatty tissue, 54 per cent of muscle, 8 per cent of bone and 2 per cent mainly tendon – what could be described as 'gristle'. In the leg, however, there will be only 22 per cent of fatty tissue but 11 per cent of bone and 6 per cent tendon, with the rest muscle. Fat is one of the most significant components of meat to affect the esteem with which it is held by consumers. Generally speaking, there is an ideal amount of fat as well as an ideal distribution. There can be too much or there can be too little for a joint of meat to be judged as being of the highest quality. Fat may be laid down between the muscle fibres and, as subcutaneous fat, under the skin. The layer of subcutaneous fat is particularly important because it prevents the meat from drying out. Because such layers tend to become thinner towards the ends of an animal's legs, animal geneticists actually breed to obtain meat-producing animals with especially short legs so that the degree of fattening between the loin and the leg may be more uniform.

Fat is deposited in various parts of an animal's body other than the muscle, where 'marbling' fat is prized for its desirable influence on the texture of the meat. The internal fat deposited round the kidneys is equally nutritious but does not add to the 'quality' of meat. It is usually cut off and converted into suet. Nor is fat appreciated when it occurs in thick layers.

In many animals used for meat, fat has a further function. It is an indication of the age of the animal and of the kind of life it has led. The age of all animals is reflected, as I have already pointed out, in the conformation of their body and hence – if they are to be eaten – in the character of their meat. The colour of the fat may also indicate the age of the animal. If a butcher sees that the fat in a side of beef is darkly coloured he can conclude that the orange pigment from the grass it has eaten has accumulated in it. If the beast has subsequently suffered a period of poor feeding, it will have consumed part of its own fat and the pigment will have become concentrated in what remains. It follows that cows and old animals usually have darker coloured fat than young animals which have been specially fattened for meat.

Colour and flavour The colour of muscle also is an indication of the history of the animal from which it comes. The function of the muscle haemoglobin is to sustain activity. Darker coloured muscles containing more haemoglobin are, therefore, those which are most vigorously exercised. The muscles of hares and other game animals tend to be darker than those of domesticated rabbits which lead more sedentary lives. Young calves and stock which are confined while they are being fattened have paler muscular tissues than those found in bulls. Horsemeat is particularly darkly coloured. There is also a difference in the colour of different muscles in the same animal. The *extensor pedis* muscle in a sheep which functions continuously to keep the animal standing up is darkly coloured while the *semi-tendinosus* which is only occasionally used is much lighter. These occur together in a leg of mutton which is, in scientific terms, a mixture of anatomical structures.

The presence of colour, indicative of age and muscular activity in the animal, is also associated with more pronounced flavour in the meat. And since there is an optimum flavour at which meat is

2·2 Photomicrograph of muscle in transverse section to show muscle fibres arranged in bundles. The density of fibres per bundle and the size of the bundles affect the quality of meat.

deemed to be most desirable, colour scales have been produced for judging the quality of meat. Too pale meat may be considered to be insipid whereas very darkly coloured meat may be thought to be too strongly flavoured. Although the flavour and smell of meat do not of themselves affect its main composition and its consequent value as food, they very directly influence its acceptability. The substances which are responsible for smell and taste are often present in a food in very small concentration. A great deal of recent study is being devoted to these compounds, but knowledge of their composition is still incomplete. It is, however, clear that the physiological state of an animal may very significantly affect the taste and smell of its meat. A striking example upon which much research is being done is pork.

The smell of sex The muscle and particularly the fat of certain adult male pigs are known to develop a nauseating smell when they are heated. This so-called 'boar odour' may be so powerful as to render the meat effectively uneatable. It appears that the substances causing this taint, a mixture including the compound, p-cresol, are concerned with the sexual activity of the animals and may act as attractants to pigs of the opposite sex. The 'boar odour' has been found to be present in concentrations sufficient to diminish or destroy the quality of the meat as acceptable human food in 64 per cent of the boars tested and also in 5 per cent of virgin females and castrated males. While this phenomenon is most strikingly seen in pigs, its existence represents as a general principle a further respect in which the state and activity of an animal may influence the meat derived from it.

Meat texture The texture of meat, like its flavour, is another factor which, although of little significance to its nutritional value and affecting its chemical composition not at all, is also of very great importance to those who judge quality. Here again, the physiological activity of the animal exerts a marked influence. The texture of muscle, and thus the eating qualities of the meat, depends

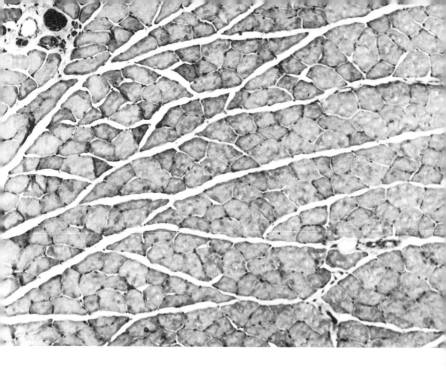

on the grain and size of the 'bundles' within the muscle. In large animals such as cattle these bundles are larger than in smaller animals – sheep and pigs, for example. Similarly, the texture of different muscles within the same animal differs. Within a single leg of mutton, the *gracilis* is very much finer in grain than the *vastus* muscle. The anatomical structure of muscle and its texture are shown in figure 2·2.

The chemical composition of meat The protein of meat provides it with its main physical characteristics, as it also does with its dietetic and nutritional properties. Nevertheless, meat may also contain large and variable amounts of fat. Some meat also contains carbo-hydrate, mainly in the form of the storage starch-like substance, glycogen. The main components of different types of meat and meat from various animals are shown in table 2·1. The figures set out in table 2·1 illustrate clearly that the main difference in composition between meat from different sources depends on the amount of fat. The values given in the table can only be taken as

Table 2·1 Composition of various meats (per 100 g of edible material)

		Water	Kilo calories	Protein	Fat	Carbohydrate
		%		g	g	g
Bacon		19·3	665	8·4	69·3	1·0
Beef	carcase	60·3	263	18·5	20·4	0
	rib	51·7	352	16·2	31·4	0
	steak	49·1	380	15·5	34·8	0
Brains	beef, pig or sheep	78·9	125	10·4	8·6	0·8
Chicken	light meat	73·7	117	23·4	1·9	0
	dark meat	73·7	130	20·6	4·7	0
Duck	domestic	54·3	326	16·0	28·6	0
	wild	61·1	233	21·1	15·8	0
Goose	domestic	51·1	354	16·4	31·5	0
Heart	beef	77·5	108	17·1	3·6	0·7
	lamb	71·6	162	16·8	9·6	1·0
	pig	77·4	113	16·8	4·4	0·4
Kidney	beef	75·9	130	15·4	6·7	0·9
	lamb	77·7	105	16·8	3·3	0·9
	pig	77·8	106	16·3	3·6	1·1
Lamb	leg	60·8	262	16·9	21·0	0
	loin	52·0	351	14·7	32·0	0
	shoulder	55·9	318	14·7	28·3	0
Liver	beef	69·7	140	19·9	3·8	5·3
	lamb	70·8	136	21·0	3·9	2·9
	pig	71·6	131	20·6	3·7	2·6
Pork	carcase	33·4	553	9·1	57·1	0
	loin	57·2	298	17·1	24·9	0
Rabbit	domestic	70·0	162	21·0	8·0	0
	wild	73·0	135	21·0	5·0	0
Reindeer	side	63·3	217	20·5	14·4	0
	forequarter	67·4	178	21·8	9·4	0
	hindquarter	59·6	256	19·4	19·2	0
Sweetbreads (thymus)	beef	67·8	207	14·6	16·0	0
	lamb	79·5	94	14·1	3·8	0
Tongue	beef	68·0	207	16·4	15·0	0·4
	lamb	69·5	199	13·9	15·3	0·5
	pig	66·1	215	16·8	15·6	0·5
Tripe	beef	79·1	100	19·1	2·0	0
Veal	loin	69·0	181	19·2	11·0	0
Venison		74·0	126	21·0	4·0	0
Whale		70·9	156	20·6	7·5	0

Calcium	Phosphorus	Iron	Vitamin A	Thiamine	Riboflavin	Niacin	Ascorbic acid
mg	mg	mg	iu	mg	mg	mg	mg
13	108	1·2	0	0·36	0·11	1·8	0
11	171	2·8	40	0·08	0·16	4·4	0
9	148	2·4	60	0·07	0·14	3·9	0
9	142	2·3	70	0·07	0·14	3·7	0
10	312	2·4	0	0·23	0·26	4·4	18
11	218	1·1	60	0·05	0·09	10·7	0
13	188	1·5	150	0·08	0·20	5·2	0
10	176	1·6	0	0·08	0·19	6·7	0
10	176	1·6	0	0·08	0·19	6·7	0
5	195	4·0	20	0·53	0·88	7·5	2
14	231		100	0·21	1·03	6·4	trace
3	131	3·3	30	0·43	1·24	6·6	3
11	219	7·4	690	0·36	2·55	6·4	15
13	218	7·6	690	0·51	2·42	7·4	15
11	218	6·7	130	0·58	1·73	9·8	12
10	152	1·3	0	0·15	0·21	4·9	0
9	127	1·0	0	0·13	0·18	4·3	0
9	127	1·0	0	0·13	0·18	4·3	0
8	352	6·5	43,900	0·25	3·26	13·6	31
10	349	10·9	50,500	0·40	3·28	16·9	33
10	356	19·2	10,900	0·30	3·03	16·4	23
5	88	1·4	0	0·44	0·10	2·4	0
10	193	2·6	0	0·83	0·20	4·4	0
20	352	1·3	0	0·08	0·06	12·8	0
8	182	2·1	0	0·12	0·29	5·0	0
29	186	1·4	0	0·07	0·29	3·5	0
127	86	1·6	0		0·15	1·6	0
11	195	2·9	0	0·14	0·26	6·4	0
10	249		0	0 23	0·48	6·3	0
12	144		1,860	0·09	0·08		6

representative. For example, although the selected figure for the fat in leg of lamb is 21·0 per cent, values significantly less, say, 14 per cent are commonly found or, on the other hand, values substantially greater. This can easily be understood in the light of the factors affecting the growth of the animal which have been discussed. The fluctuation in fat content directly influences the calorific value of the meat since each gram of fat contributes 9 kilocalories whereas an equal weight of protein only contributes 4 kilocalories. All the components of meat are of course inversely proportional to the water content, which tends to diminish as the animal becomes older. When meats are considered as a group, excluding the glandular organs such as liver and kidney, it can be seen that after making allowance for the fluctuations in fat and moisture, the other components, that is calcium, phosphorous and iron, and the several vitamins are present, as might be expected, in broadly similar amounts. Whale meat is, however, exceptional in containing large amounts of vitamin A derived from the marine diet of the animal from which it is derived.

The composition of heart differs in some respects from that of other meat as does that of brains and kidney. Liver, however, differs most strikingly. Because it serves as a storage organ for certain of the nutrients consumed by an animal in excess of its current needs, it contains substantial concentrations of vitamins, particularly vitamin A. But it is also rich in the B-vitamins, thiamine, riboflavin and niacin, and in iron. A noteworthy feature of heart, brains, kidney and liver is that they contain significant amounts of vitamin C. Usually this is unimportant because vitamin C is mainly derived from fruit and vegetables and meat provides protein as its principal contribution to the diet. Under certain circumstances, however, the vitamin C-content may be crucial.

There have been several examples of people in the Arctic surviving and remaining free from scurvy (the disease which occurs when insufficient vitamin C is available) provided they ate an ample quantity of fresh meat. We know that the Norwegian explorers, Nansen and Johanson, after leaving their ship, the *Fram*,

spent nine months including the winter of 1895–6 on Frederick
Jackson Island and remained free from scurvy, although obtaining
no lemon juice or fresh vegetables and subsisting mainly on fresh
walrus and bear meat. Two other travellers, Jackson and Harley,
described in 1900 an interesting incident at Kharborova in the
Yugor Straits. Six Russian priests arrived in the autumn attended
by a small Russian boy. The priests were prevented by their
religious vows from eating fresh meat and were, therefore, com-
pelled to subsist as long as they were able on salt fish. The boy ate
fresh reindeer meat throughout the winter. When spring came the
following May, he was the only one alive, all of his masters having
died of scurvy.

The food value of meat The value of meat as food must, like almost
every article of diet, be considered from several aspects. The first is
nutritional. As an item of a conventional Western diet, meat makes a
valuable contribution of protein. Rather, since almost every diet in
an industrial society, except that of the very poorest people, almost
always contains sufficient protein, it is more accurate to consider
meat as contributing *amino acids*, and particularly the amino acid,
lysine, of which shortage is most probable. Table 2·2 shows the
amino acid make-up of a number of proteins from different sources
assessed in relation to their nutritional value. There are in living
tissues numerous proteins which differ from each other in a number
of subtle respects. For example, it is recognised that skin trans-
plants can be transferred only from one identical twin to another.
Individuals reject from their tissues 'foreign' proteins because they
differ in some subtle degree one from another. Yet although
proteins of obviously different structure are markedly different in
amino acid composition, in general the proteins when eaten –
that is, when used as human food – are all approximately equal in
value.

   The second component of meat that is of nutritional significance
is fat. The composition of fat and its consequent texture is affected
partly by the food eaten by the animal concerned, partly by the

Table 2·2 Food value of protein from different sources in terms of their essential amino acid composition (mg amino acid/g nitrogen)

	Iso-leucine	Leucine	Lysine⁻	Phenylalanine
'Ideal' protein	270	306	270	180
Egg	428	565	396	368
Meat (beef)	332	515	540	256
Milk (cows)	407	630	496	311
Fish	317	474	549	231
Oats	302	436	212	309
Rice	322	535	236	307
Flour (white)	262	442	126	322
Cassava	118	184	310	133

temperature of the environment and partly by the species of animal. When we talk about fat in an animal – or person, for that matter – we really refer to adipose tissue. This consists of diffuse connective tissue in which the cells have become loaded with droplets of fat. Abdominal fat, which is laid down within the abdominal cavity where the temperature is comparatively warm, is harder and melts at a higher temperature than the superficial fat on, for example, the animal's back, where the temperature is slightly cooler. The different consistency of fat from, say, a pig, a sheep and a goose is reflected in its chemical composition. Differences can also be produced by feeding. For example, if too much cod-liver oil is included in a pig's ration, its fat will be contaminated. In spite of all these differences, however, there is little or no difference in the nutritional value of different meat fats.

Reference has already been made to the fat-soluble vitamin A found in liver and some other meats. This and the B-vitamins, notably niacin and also cyanocobalamin (vitamin B_{12}) which is also present, make meat a food of nutritional significance.

It is, perhaps, worth discussing the difference between the chemistry of muscle as it is in the body of the living animal and that of the meat which it becomes after the beast is killed. When a well-fed animal is lying resting in a stall or standing quietly in a field

Tyrosine	Methionine	Threonine	Typtophan	Valine	Protein score
180	144	180	90	270	100
274	196	310	106	460	100
212	154	275	75	345	83
323	154	292	90	440	78
159	178	283	62	327	70
213	84	192	74	348	79
269	142	241	65	415	72
174	78	174	69	262	47
98	22	136	131	144	22

there is in its muscles about 1 per cent of glycogen. This is sometimes termed 'animal starch'. In an active animal the glycogen is
broken down, first to glucose, and then, through a series of linked
biochemical reactions, partly to lactic acid and partly to carbon
dioxide. This is the process by which muscular energy is released.
When rested, well-fed animals are killed, this chain of reactions is
set off. The lactic acid produced gives a certain natural acidity to
the meat in which it acts as a preservative. If, on the other hand, the
animal is fasted before being killed or if it has undergone an arduous
journey to the abbatoir or has struggled before being slaughtered,
or even if it has been made to stand restlessly or been frightened,
the glycogen in its muscles becomes depleted and, in consequence,
the acidity cannot build up in the meat. This lack of acidity, while
it has little immediate effect on the nutritional value of the meat,
damages its aesthetic value in several ways and, to that extent,
reduces its quality as food. First of all, the lactic acid in the meat
from animals killed while the level of glycogen in their muscles is
high prevents bacterial infection. But a second effect which has been
recognised since as long ago as the eighteenth century is that meat
from exhausted and frightened animals exhibits the aesthetically
unpleasant phenomenon of 'dark-cutting' in beef or, in pigs,
'glazy' bacon.

What is muscle in life, which becomes meat after death, is made up of a variety of components. There are myofibrils which together form the individual muscle fibres. These are composed of the proteins, myosin, tropomyosin, so called X-protein, and actin. Between the separate muscle fibres is a juice called the sarcoplasm in which are found a group of chemically different proteins, myogen and globulins. There is also a fine network of tubules between the fibres; these constitute the sarcoplasmic reticulum in which the protein, elastin, occurs. The muscle fibres themselves are encased in a thin membrane, the sarcolemma, by which they are attached to the tough connective tissue through which the pull of the muscle is exerted. The whole of this complex system by which a living creature is enabled to move is in life kept supplied by the blood stream with oxygen for its biochemical activity and, dissolved in the muscle juice, are various compounds including the glycogen, glucose and glucose phosphates which constitute the fuel upon which the muscles operate and lactic acid the partially used fuel, together with creatine, inosine monophosphate, phospho-pyridine nucleotides, amino acids and the bases, carnosine and anserine – all these in a state of dynamic equilibrium. As soon as the animal is killed and its blood ceases to flow and bring in oxygen and take away breakdown products of metabolism the equilibrium is destroyed. One of the most obvious effects is a change in the structure of the myofibrillar proteins, myosin, tropomyocin, X-protein and actin, causing them to exude water. Sarcoplasmic proteins myogen, globulin and myoglobin, may partially break down into their component amino acids which, apart from changing the composition of the muscle mass, provides a rich medium for bacteria. To avoid as far as possible the aesthetically undesirable effects of these changes, the butcher takes pains to bleed the animal as soon as he has killed it as quickly and completely as possible.

We thus come to the fact that the appearance of meat from an animal properly bled after slaughter is an important criterion in the assessment of its food value. Secondly, the structure of the meat and particularly the extent to which the muscle proteins have lost

glycine

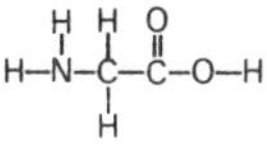

alanine

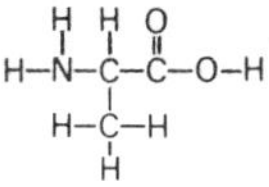

valine

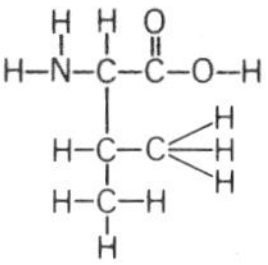

isoleucine

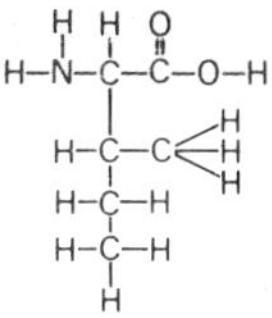

$$H-N-C-C-O-H$$

leucine

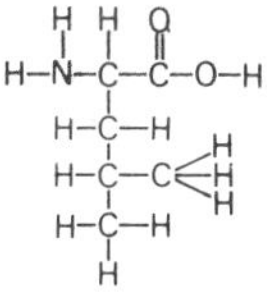

lycine

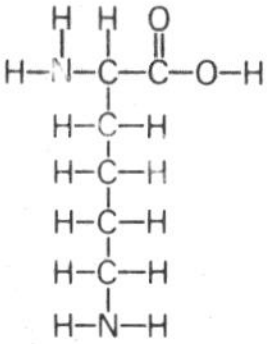

arginine

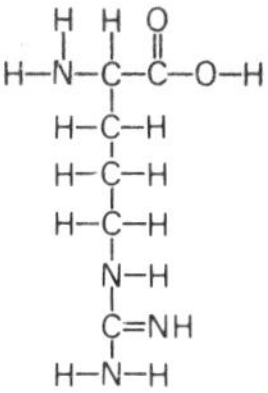

histidine

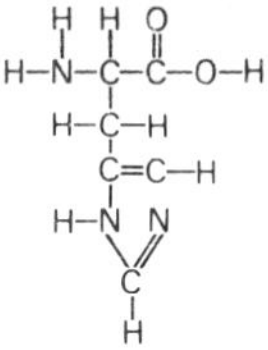

proline

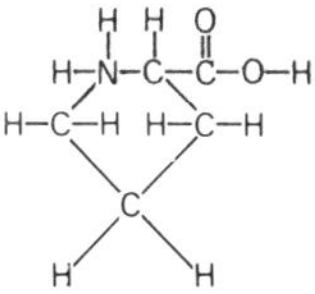

hydroxyproline

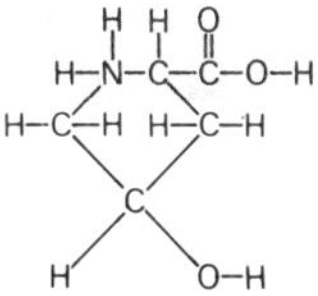

serine

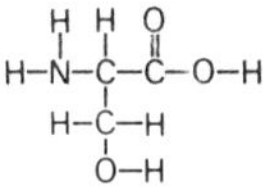

threonine

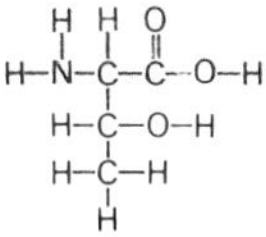

aspartic acid

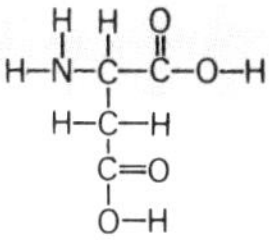

glutamic acid

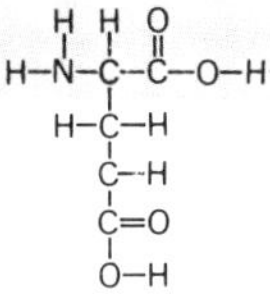

tyrosine

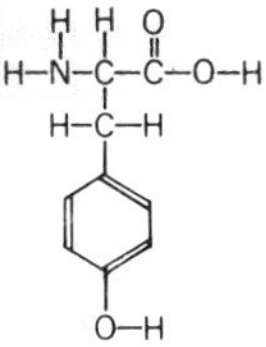

cysteine

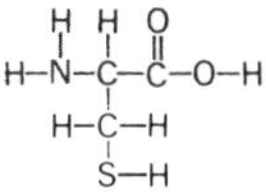

methionine

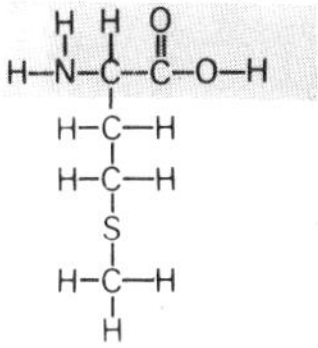

cystine

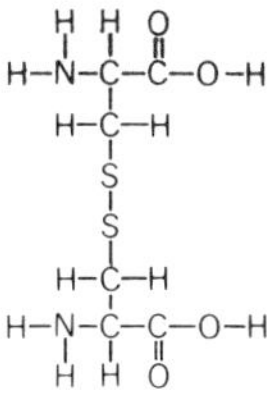

tryptophan

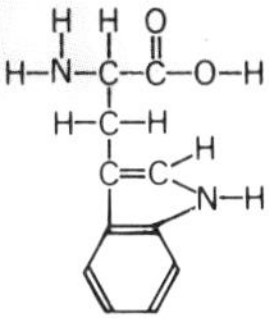

phenylalanine

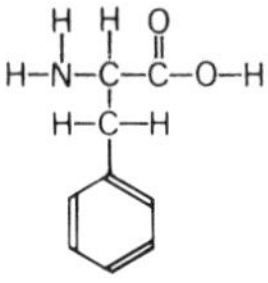

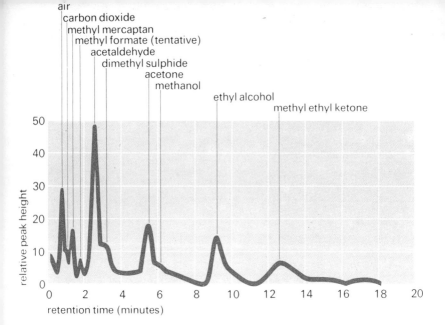

air
carbon dioxide
methyl mercaptan
methyl formate (tentative)
acetaldehyde
dimethyl sulphide
acetone
methanol
ethyl alcohol
methyl ethyl ketone

relative peak height

retention time (minutes)

the water which is an integral part of their molecular composition in life, is also important. Thirdly, however, there is the taste and aroma of the meat when cooked. The amount of such compounds as carnosine and anserine, of nucleotides and of other so-called 'extractives', the action of micro-organisms, the presence of rancidity in the meat fat – all these affect taste. Aroma, equally or more importantly, is a topic of intense current research which has still far to go before a clear solution is reached. Figure 2·4, for example, shows the complexity of the combination of substances, many present in extremely small concentration, which are associated with the aroma of meat.

It is a remarkable fact that in spite of the general similarity of the food value, taste and chemical composition of meat from different species of animals, the number of species used at all widely is small. Cattle, sheep and pigs dominate the local consumption and international trade of the industrial nations of the world. Long-continued breeding has produced strains which yield a much greater return in human food for each unit weight of feed provided for the

2·4 An analysis of the smell of meat. The various compounds have been separated by the analytical technique of gas chromatography. Almost certainly these are not all the components which give meat its distinctive aroma.

29

animal than is obtainable from unimproved or wild varieties. Meat animals can be thought of as machines for concentrating plant nutrients and converting them into palatable and nutritious meat or milk. On this basis, it can be calculated that, on average, for each 100 parts of feed energy (in terms of kilocalories) fed to it, a pig returns 20 per cent as pork, a cow gives back 15 per cent as milk, a hen 7 per cent as eggs and a chicken 5 per cent as flesh. Finally, for each 100 units of feed energy consumed, an ox and a sheep both yield 4 energy units of meat. The conversion of vegetable protein from feed into meat protein is of similar efficiency. Again, cows and pigs return most: for every 100 g of protein feed, 14·5 g of protein are recovered as milk and pork. Poultry are nearly as efficient: they return an average of 13·5 g. Ox and sheep return 8·5 g and 4·5 g.

But these calculations are not altogether meaningful. Although a sheep pastured on a high hillside accumulates comparatively little of what it eats for human consumption, without it the human community would gain no food at all. In fact, a sheep can utilise steep and rocky land from which alternative crops and, particularly, crops of food of such high aesthetic excellence and nutritional value as meat, could not be obtained. This makes it doubly interesting that so restricted a number of animal species are eaten.

The selection of one type of animal as a source of meat and the rejection of another has little to do with the food value of the meat. Horse-meat in general contains less fat than beef but this is only partly due to the species and habits of the animal. It is due to an almost equal extent to the fact that improved breeds of cattle, but not of horses, have been developed specially for meat and that cattle, but not horses, are specially fattened for market. Horse-flesh, though not much eaten in Europe or the Americas and specifically avoided in Ethiopia, is quite commonly employed for food in an extensive area of the less industrialised parts of north-central Asia. In the same way, pork, while widely consumed in Europe, America and other industrialised countries is rigidly avoided in the Islamic parts of the world, notably the Middle East, in certain parts of Africa, particularly East Africa, and in some of the more remote

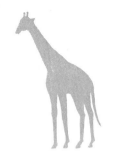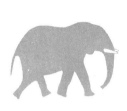

	giraffe	elephant
environment	open forest	open forest, rain forest, marshes
feeding habits	browses treetops, high shrubbery	browses, breaks down forest
adaptability to harvesting	good	excellent
equivalent to	40 sheep	80 sheep

republics of the Soviet Union. Beef as well, though a popular meat in the West and in many other places, is rigidly avoided in India. Finally, it is interesting to note that although both the pig and the dog were among the earliest animals to be domesticated by man and used both as scavengers and for food, both are rejected with equal horror by particular human groups in modern times. While dog-flesh is never used for meat by the industrialised nations of the world, it is a popular article of diet in Borneo, New Guinea and most of the island archipelagos of the Pacific, in considerable areas of eastern Asia and in many of the countries of central West Africa.

In recent years, thought has been given to the best way to extend the present restricted list of animals used as a source of meat. Since the refusal of different national groups to eat the meat of particular animals is based on deeply rooted ethnological causes, rather than concentrate on ways of breaking down these human prejudices, study has been made of the feasibility of making use of the meat of

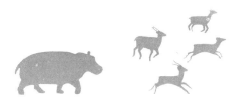

2·5 Some animals which could be used for meat. There is no reason why only beef, mutton and pork should maintain a virtual monopoly of the market.

hippopotamus	antelope
all rivers and lakes	open forest, savanna
eats water plants	browses and grazes
excellent	excellent
60 sheep	3-12 sheep

animals at present not seen in the international food market at all. For example, there are large areas of the African continent which appear to be basically unsuited to farming, from which substantial crops of wild animals could be harvested for meat. Among these are the giraffe, elephant, hippopotamus and more than twenty varieties of antelope. The environment inhabited by these animals, their feeding habits, adaptability to harvesting, and food-equivalent when compared with sheep are shown diagrammatically in figure 2·5. All these animals are capable of living in territory unsuitable for conventional animal husbandry and eating fodder which is unsuitable either as human food or as feed for other animals.

Among other animals at present neglected by food producers but which could well be utilised for meat, the freshwater manatee, *Sirenia*, has been particularly singled out. The manatee, together with the marine dugong, are herbivores which are entirely aquatic. They feed on water plants which are neglected by other livestock and whose removal may indeed be beneficial in keeping waterways clear. The yield of meat for each pound of feed consumed by these animals is higher than that often obtained from conventional livestock.

The trend in modern scientific food production for the number of animal species to be continuously reduced – that is to say, for local breeds to be superseded by stock imported from comparatively few specialised centres – may lead to improved productivity in parts of the world where the environmental conditions are comparatively uniform. To try to import European or North American stock into Africa or Asia may, however, be mistaken and unscientific. It is only logical to recognise that animals which evolved in a particular area should be better adapted to it than animals only recently introduced. In 1950, a survey carried out in Kenya showed that the live-weight of animals capable of subsisting in an area was often greater when it was made up of wild animals than when domestic livestock were specially introduced for meat. Indeed, in parts infested by the tsetse fly domesticated animals cannot be reared at all. The figures are striking. In the Kenya Highlands, up to 32,000 lb weight of cattle can be supported on a square mile of territory. But in the savanna country of Masailand, from 70,000 to 100,000 lb of mixed wild ungulates can live on each square mile. And in bush country where the tsetse flies prevent any cattle living, the land can support 30,000 lb of wild ungulates.

An important reason why more meat can be produced from a unit area of land in the form of wild animals than of domestic cattle is that the diets of the different animals are complementary to each other. They either eat different food plants or eat plants at different stages of their growth. The result of these non-duplicating food preferences is that virtually all of the herbage can be used to support one kind of livestock or another, whereas when merely sheep or cattle or even goats are kept, only one kind of crop – usually grass – is eaten and much of the rest left.

It is interesting to note that wild creatures produce meat as efficiently as cattle bred for the purpose. If we assume that beef cattle increase in weight by an average of 0·30 lb per day and sheep by 0·12 lb per day, the growth rate of wild African ungulates is just as fast or even faster.

These wild animals reach marketable age just as quickly as domestic livestock kept under conditions of good management, and give more meat. The 'killing-out' weight of the majority of African-owned cattle seldom exceeds 50 per cent of the live-weight. On the other hand, the killing-out weight of Grant's gazelle has been shown to be 63 per cent, that of impalas and elands 59 per cent, Thomson's gazelles 57 per cent, topis and konegonis 53 per cent, and wildebeests an average of 51 per cent.

The problem of cropping wild animals for meat has already been solved. Free ranging animals can be most conveniently shot at night. Even large animals such as elephants have been successfully slaughtered in this way, bled and transported back to a central abattoir. Game meat, including hippopotamus, has been canned and has found ready acceptance among Europeans and Americans. Perhaps most promising of all developments for the future have been the successful examples of the domestication of wild animals for meat production. This was done in neolithic times, according

Table 2·3 Approximate daily liveweight gain (lb) of wild ungulates on east and central African ranges

Eland (*Torotragus buselaphus*)	0·73
Wildebeest (*Gorgon taurinus*)	0·52–0·41
Kongoni (*Alcelaphus buselaphus*)	0·50–0·39
Topi (*Damaliscus lunatus*)	0·44–0·34
Grant's gazelle (*Gazella* sp.)	0·26–0·22
Impala (*Aepyceros melampus*)	0·26–0·20
Thomson's gazelle (*Gazella* sp.)	0·13–0·08

to the evidence of cave paintings and of kitchen refuse, but was later abandoned. Now there is a successful 'domestic' herd of eland in Rhodesia which is handled and herded in the same manner as domestic cattle.

Before concluding this section, I ought to refer briefly to the whale. This animal has provided very large quantities of fat for human food, and particularly since highly mechanised systems of killing whales and processing them at sea have been developed, whale oil, used largely for the manufacture of margarine, has formed a major commodity of international trade. Much of the meat, however, has been wasted. In spite of possessing nutritional value approximately equal to that of meat from other sources, it has never attained the same esteem as food. This has been due to the fact that the fat in whale meat possesses a characteristic 'fishy' flavour which is unattractive to most consumers. There has, therefore, not been sufficient incentive to whalers to make it worth their while, in economic terms, to preserve the meat over the long distances from the ocean to the world markets and to attempt to popularise the meat. Recently, inadequate control over the highly efficient technological killing methods make it possible that at least some species of whales will become extinct before long.

Fish

It is interesting to note that fish, which were the first wild creatures to be hunted for food, still remain after more than forty thousand years of human history the last wild beast to be pursued and captured as a major article of diet. The refuse of shellfish has been found in the kitchen middens of the most ancient sites of human habitations. Far inland, the bones of sea fish were discovered in the refuse heaps of the late Old Stone Age cave dwellers in the Dordogne, dating from about 40,000 BC.

The food value of fish, like that of meat, is determined by the balance between the amounts of protein, fat and water present in their flesh. The proportion of fat, and the correspondingly affected amount of protein, are mainly influenced by the species of the fish. Sea fish can be divided into two groups, the *pelagic* fish, which live in the middle and surface layers of the water, and the *demersal* fish, which inhabit the bottom of the sea. Pelagic fish, which include herring and mackerel, feed on plankton which grows in the sea much as pasture crops grow on land. Demersal fish, which include cod, haddock, whiting and flat fish, while they are young also eat plankton; later, however, they prey on crabs and other crustacea and then on small fish such as herrings and sprats. The pelagic fish contain up to 20 per cent of fat while the demersal fish contain very little fat. Cod, haddock and whiting, which are among the most important species as a source of human food, contain only 0·5 per cent of fat and are, in consequence, excellent sources of protein. Among other demersal fish, plaice, megrim, lemon sole and bass may contain about 2 per cent of fat, and halibut, mullet and dogfish up to 5 per cent.

The composition of fish of single species, again like the composition of meat, depends on a number of physiological factors. Perhaps the most important is the sexual state of the fish. Herrings, for example, may contain 20 per cent of fat in July and only 8 per cent in April.

The food value of fish can readily be seen to be made up of two components. First is its nutritional value. This is in almost every respect equal to that of meat. The proportion of the total energy value of the flesh of cod, bass, albacore, flounder and haddock derived from the protein in it exceeds 90 per cent, whereas in lean meat it is only 60 per cent. A variety of tests on animals and human beings has demonstrated the biological value of fish protein to be superior to that of the protein in milk. The amino acid content of a number of varieties of fish compared with that of meat is shown in table 2·4. The composition of many of the principal food fishes is shown in table 2·5. Yet in spite of its high nutritional value, the value in terms of esteem which people put upon fish is frequently less than that given to meat.

Fish, of course, is highly perishable. Two reasons why fish goes

Table 2·4 Composition of fish (per 100 g edible material)

	Water	Kilo-calories	Protein	Fat	Carbo-hydrate
	%		g	g	g
Barracuda	75·4	113	21·0	2·6	0
Bass black	79·3	93	19·2	1·2	0
white	78·8	98	18·0	2·3	0
Bluefish	75·4	117	20·5	3·3	0
Bonito	67·6	168	24·0	7·3	0
Clams	85·8	54	8·6	1·0	2·0
Cod	81·2	78	17·6	0·3	0
Crab	78·5	93	17·3	1·9	0·5
Dogfish	72·3	156	17·6	9·0	0
Flatfish (flounder, sole)	81·3	79	16·7	0·8	0
Haddock	80·5	79	18·3	0·1	0
Hake	81·8	74	16·5	0·4	0
Halibut	76·5	100	20·9	1·2	0
Herring	69·0	176	17·3	11·3	0
Mackerel	67·2	191	19·0	12·2	0
Mullet	72·6	146	19·6	6·9	0
Oysters	84·6	66	8·4	1·8	3·4
Perch	75·7	118	19·3	4·0	0
Pike	78·8	90	19·1	0·9	0
Pollock	77·4	95	20·4	0·9	0
Salmon	63·6	217	22·5	13·4	0
Sardine	70·7	160	19·2	8·6	0
Scollop	79·8	81	15·3	0·2	3·3
Shad	70·4	170	18·6	10·0	0
Shrimp	78·2	91	18·1	0·8	1·5
Skate	77·8	98	21·5	0·7	0
Squid	80·2	84	16·4	0·9	1·5
Sturgeon	78·7	94	18·1	1·9	0
Swordfish	75·9	118	19·2	4·0	0
Trout	66·3	195	21·5	11·4	0
Tuna	70·5	145	25·2	4·1	0
Whiting	77·3	105	18·3	3·0	0

Cal-cium	Phos-phorus	Iron	Vitamin A	Thiamine	Ribo-flavin	Niacin	Ascorbic acid
mg	mg	mg	iu	mg	mg	mg	mg
—	—	—	—	—	—	—	—
—	—	—	—	—	—	—	—
—	—	—	—	—	—	—	—
23	243	0·6	—	0·12	0·09	1·9	—
—	—	—	—	—	—	—	—
—	208	—	—	—	—	—	—
10	194	0·4	0	0·06	0·07	2·2	2
43	175	0·8	2,170	0·16	0·08	2·8	2
—	—	—	—	0·05	—	—	—
12	195	0·8	0	0·05	0·05	1·7	—
23	197	0·7	0	0·04	0·07	3·0	—
41	142	—	0	0·10	0·20	—	—
13	211	0·7	440	0·07	0·07	8·3	—
—	256	1·1	110	0·02	0·15	3·6	—
5	239	1·0	450	0·15	0·33	8·2	—
26	220	1·8	—	0·07	0·08	5·2	—
94	143	5·5	310	0·14	0·18	2·5	—
—	192	—	—	—	—	—	—
—	—	—	—	—	—	—	—
—	—	—	—	0·05	0·10	1·6	—
79	186	0·9	310	0·10	0·23	7·2	9
33	215	1·8	—	—	—	—	—
26	208	1·8	—	—	0·06	1·3	—
20	260	0·5	—	0·15	0·24	8·4	—
63	166	1·6	—	0·02	0·03	3·2	—
—	—	—	—	0·02	—	—	—
12	119	0·5	—	0·02	0·12	—	—
—	—	—	—	—	—	—	—
19	195	0·9	1,580	0·05	0·05	8·0	—
—	—	—	—	0·08	0·20	8·4	—
—	—	—	—	—	—	—	—
—	—	—	—	—	—	—	—

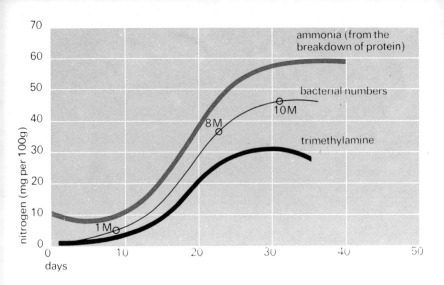

Table 2·5 Average amino acid content of fish and meat samples* (values given as per cent of protein, N × 6·25)

Essential amino acids	Atlantic mackerel	Pacific mackerel	Atlantic sardine	Pacific sardine
	(6)†	(6)	(6)	(8)
Arginine	5·8	5·5	5·5	5·1
Histidine	3·8	5·4	2·4	4·7
Isoleucine	5·2	5·0	4·0	4·6
Leucine	7·2	7·4	7·1	7·2
Lysine	8·1	8·5	7·8	8·4
Methionine	2·7	2·8	2·7	2·8
Phenylalanine	3·5	3·8	3·4	3·7
Threonine	4·9	4·5	4·4	4·3
Tryptophan	1·0	1·0	0·8	1·0
Valine	5·4	5·2	5·0	5·2

2·6 The graph shows the increase in bacterial numbers and the corresponding increase in trimethylamine and ammonia in haddock stored in ice as it gradually becomes 'stale'.

39

bad so quickly is, first, that because it is not possible to stop fish struggling before they die, the glycogen from their muscles becomes depleted and lactic acid is not therefore released to act as a preservative. The second reason is that fish flesh contains between 0·2 and 2·0 per cent of a nitrogenous compound, trimethylamine oxide. When the fish dies, bacteria break down this substance into trimethylamine, which contributes to the characteristically unattractive smell of bad fish. The progress of this chemical breakdown is illustrated in figure 2·6. Perhaps, therefore, the fact that some of the fish marketed has started to go stale has damaged its reputation

Atlantic herring‡	Salmon	Tuna	Beef	Whole ham
	(6)	(8)	(2)	(4)
7·1	5·8	6·4	5·3	6·1
1·9	2·6	3·5	5·7	3·6
6·2	4·9	4·9	4·7	5·0
7·1	7·3	7·9	7·2	7·8
8·3	8·0	8·9	8·3	8·7
2·6	3·0	2·5	2·8	2·7
3·6	3·7	3·8	3·5	3·8
4·1	4·4	4·2	4·5	4·5
0·8	0·9	1·0	1·0	1·0
5·4	5·6	5·4	5·1	5·2

* Sources: Neilands et al. 1949
† Figures in parentheses in column headings indicate number of samples
‡ Data for Atlantic herring from Boge 1960

as an attractive food, particularly in industrialised communities.

Fish is an article of diet of high nutritional value. It already makes a major contribution to human diet and, as means for developing fish farming progress further, it will become more important still. Nevertheless, it can serve as a warning against intellectual arrogance. Some fish and shellfish have from time to time been found to contain harmful substances, so called 'biotoxins', which are not always destroyed by cooking. These are quite different from bacterial toxins or food poisoning due to the presence of pathological micro-organisms. For example, 'fugu' is an intoxication which occurs from time to time, particularly in Japan, when puffers, also called globefish, *Liosaccus* sp., are eaten. The exact cause of this is still not fully understood. Paralytic shellfish poisoning has occurred in North America, Japan and elsewhere and again, although much study has been given to the problem, the cause is not entirely clear. We can today claim to possess scientific knowledge enabling us to produce food more efficiently than has ever been possible before. We understand much about the chemical composition of food and of the nutritional needs of the people eating it. Nevertheless, there is even now much more to be learned.

3 Milk, cheese, butter and eggs

Considered in scientific terms, animals, when used for food, are in fact biological machines by which coarse feeds, herbage of various sorts, and cereals are converted into very much more attractive articles. Farm animals concentrate and refine the components of their diet. In nutritional terms, they convert second-class protein into protein of first-class quality. As was already shown in chapter 2, some animals are more efficient machines for the conversion of poor quality feed into high quality food than others. All animals which produce milk to feed their young do so with remarkable efficiency. It follows, therefore, that improved livestock which have been bred specially for high yield are particularly economical units for the production of nutritious human food.

Milk

One of the most remarkable features of the modern evolution of food production in the present age of ever-advancing technology is the continuous reduction in the number of animal and plant species used widely. In considering milk as food, it is generally assumed that what is meant is cow's milk. It is, therefore, of some interest to compare the composition of cow's milk with that of milk from a number of other animal species. The average figures are given in table 3·1.

It can be seen from these figures that there are wide variations in the composition of the milk produced by different animals. The proportion of protein and minerals in the milk of a particular species bears a relationship to the speed of growth of the young of that species. If we take two terrestrial animals which live in the main under temperate conditions, it can be seen that human milk contains 1·5 per cent of protein and the human infant doubles its birth weight in 180 days; sow's milk contains 6·2 per cent of protein and the piglet doubles its weight in 14 days. The reindeer, which lives in a cold climate on a specialised diet of moss, and the porpoise, which is a marine animal, are obviously exceptional.

Production of milk by the mammary gland The mammary gland is in many ways a remarkable organ. It performs a function in some respect similar to that of the kidney. It is designed to permit a large volume of blood to flow through a network of fine tubules. These tubules possess the ability of passing certain components of the blood through their walls and at the same time preventing other components from passing. In fact, it is inaccurate to write that the fine ducts, or alveoli, allow components to 'pass' through their walls. The actual milk-forming cells can more precisely be said to 'pump' glucose and fat through into the milk while holding back much of the protein and some other components, notably sodium and chlorine. The composition of a cow's blood plasma compared with that of her milk is shown in table 3·2.

The pumping effect of the cells of a cow's mammary gland can perhaps best be appreciated by the estimate which is generally accepted that some 400 to 500 litres of blood have to pass through the circulation system of the udder to produce one litre of milk. The process, chemically and physically, must be a very complicated one in order to bring about the enormous increase in the concentration of certain compounds while reducing – or, in the case of cholesterol esters, almost completely excluding – others. In spite of intensive research into the biochemistry and physiology of milk secretion during the last twenty-five years, the full details of the mechanism are still not fully understood. Nevertheless, a good deal of useful information is now available on the part played by the endocrine system in milk production.

The production of milk is, of course, one of the effects brought about by the sexual activity of the female animal. The mammary gland itself develops at the time of puberty and is in part due to the action of hormones secreted by the ovaries and the pituitary. During pregnancy, the hormone progesterone, together with pituitary hormones, causes further development of the mammary gland. The process of lactation and the composition of the milk produced during lactation have been shown to be influenced by a number of hormones which are produced in balanced amounts by several of

Table 3·1 Average composition of milk from various animal species (g/100 ml)

	Protein	Fat	Carbohydrate	Kilocalories
Human	1·5	4·0	6·8	68
Hare	1·6	0·9	7·0	42
Ass	1·7	1·2	6·9	45
Mare	2·0	1·2	5·8	42
Mule	2·6	1·9	5·7	54
Elephant	3·5	20·6	7·3	228
Cow	3·5	3·5	5·0	66
Goat	3·7	4·8	4·5	76
Llama	3·9	3·1	5·6	66
Camel	4·2	3·2	5·3	67
Buffalo	4·3	7·5	4·5	103
Yak	5·2	7·0	4·6	100
Water buffalo	6·0	12·6	3·7	152
Sow	6·2	6·8	4·0	102
Ewe	6·5	6·9	4·9	109
Cat	9·0	3·3	4·9	85
Reindeer	9·9	17·1	2·8	205
Bitch	9·9	9·3	3·1	136
Porpoise	11·2	45·8	1·3	462
Rat	11·8	14·8	2·8	192

Table 3·2 Comparative figures for some constituents of blood plasma and milk of cows (per cent)

	Plasma	Milk	Increase in milk	Decrease in milk
Water	91·0	87·40		
Glucose	0·05	4·80	×96	
Protein	7·60	3·40		$\frac{1}{2}$
Fat	0·06	3·60	×60	
Phospholipids	0·24	0·04		$\frac{1}{6}$
Cholesterol esters	0·17	trace		total
Calcium	0·01	0·12	×12	
Phosphorus	0·01	0·10	×10	
Potassium	0·03	0·15	× 5	
Sodium	0·34	0·05		$\frac{1}{7}$
Chlorine	0·35	0·11		$\frac{1}{3}$

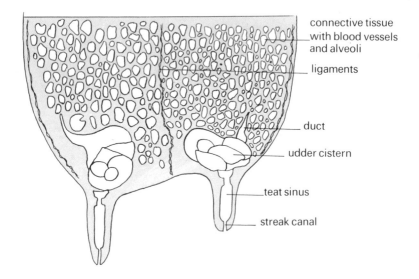

the endocrine glands. The anterior lobe of the pituitary, situated under the brain, thyroxine from the thyroid gland in the neck, cortisone from the adrenal glands close to the kidneys, and oestrogens from the ovaries all play a part.

Much more research remains to be done before the exact interaction of these hormones in the production of milk is fully understood. Already, however, existing knowledge has led to several interesting results and promises more for the future. It is known, for example, that the total amount of milk produced and the proportion of fat in it are affected by the amount of thyroxine circulating in the blood stream of the cow. This immediately raises the possibility of increasing the productivity of dairy animals should it be found feasible to supplement their natural thyroxine levels without causing undesirable side effects for example, by the injection of appropriate amounts of thyroxine. Apart from this, it has already been suggested that the increase in the butter-fat content of

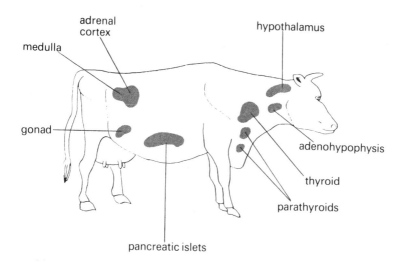

milk from cows kept under cold conditions may be due to the increase in the secretion of thyroxine, which is known to occur when the environmental temperature is reduced. It has also been suggested that the increase in the nutritional value of milk – a rise in protein, lactose and minerals – which always takes place when cows which have been kept indoors during the winter are let out in the spring may be as much due to an all-round stimulation of the endocrine system brought about by the cow's happiness in the fresh air and sunshine as to any special dietetic virtue in the new grass.

That the cow's emotions, influencing as they do the secretion of its endocrine glands, affect the production of milk has been thoroughly studied in relation to the process of milking. When the cow is soothed, by being stroked, by the suckling of a calf, or even by the playing of appropriate music in the byre, the posterior lobe of the pituitary gland secretes its hormones and milk is released by the udder. On the other hand, if the cow is roughly handled or alarmed, its adrenal glands secrete the hormone adrenaline, and the milk is held back. These examples of the intricate interplay of the various hormones explain, at least in part, the fact that although knowledge may be available to enable virgin females, or even male animals to be made to give milk by injecting them with the appropriate hormones, this procedure has so far not been developed on a practical scale.

A curious endocrine effect plays a part in the production of cow's milk in the tropics. Appetite is a more subtle physiological phenomenon than is often recognised. Many human beings, and animals as well, maintain themselves in a state of remarkable equilibrium. They eat just enough food to provide themselves with sufficient kilocalories to replace those utilised in work and the metabolic activities of the body and maintain a constant body weight – and then they stop eating. If they take more exercise and do more muscular work, they eat more, their appetite then becomes satiated and they stop eating. There are individual animals – and people – whose appetite does not 'switch off' soon enough. These become fat. The control over appetite is operated by the endocrine secretion from the hypothalamic region at the base of the brain adjacent to the pituitary. Although the control over appetite is commonly very accurate over prolonged periods of the life span, it can be put out of adjustment. For example, if the level of physical exercise falls too low, appetite control seems to become partially lost. This is the reason why beasts confined in stalls can be so readily fattened and middle-aged men who take little exercise become obese. Cows producing large quantities of milk need to maintain their appetites in order to be able to eat sufficient food to replace the nutrients expended in milk production. When cows are kept in the tropics or where the temperature is hot, their appetite-control system restricts the amount they are able to eat and in consequence their ability to produce milk is correspondingly reduced. Since the food supplies of people in tropical countries are often particularly exiguous, this physiological restriction on the

3·3 Control over appetite is maintained by the endocrine secretion of the hypothalamic region at the base of the brain, adjacent to the pituitary. This part of the brain of the left-hand rat has been experimentally damaged and the animal has become grossly obese; the right-hand rat is the normal littermate control.

efficiency of dairy cows presents a special challenge to scientific research. A dairy cow of an improved breed capable of yielding a large supply of good quality milk in an environmental temperature of 16°C will only eat a half or even a third as much food when the shade temperature is 32°C and may produce no more than 30 per cent as much milk.

The quality of the feed fed to a cow and, more particularly, the amount it eats, obviously exert an important effect on the yield and chemical composition of its milk. Typical figures for the main constituents of cow's milk are shown in table 3·3. Although certain of these constituents, for example the vitamin A-activity, are directly affected by the composition of the cow's diet, others are affected indirectly in rather a curious way. A cow is a ruminant. That is to say, while it digests a substantial proportion of the food it eats with its own digestive enzymes, it also depends for a significant proportion of its nutrition on the complex population of living creatures in its rumen. The fat in milk, so-called butter fat, possesses a peculiar and characteristic chemical composition which makes it particularly prized as an article of human diet. One of its characteristic properties is due to the presence in it of the component butyric acid. This member of the chemical group of *fatty acids* is unusual in being composed of a short chain of only four carbon

Table 3·3 Typical values for the composition of cow's milk (per 100 g)

	g		mg		iu
Water	87·4	Thiamine	0·045	Vitamin A	150
Fat	3·6	Riboflavin	0·150	Carotene	
Lactose	4·8	Niacin	0·080		
Protein	3·4	Pantothenic acid	0·300		
Calcium	0·125	Inositol	18·000		
Phosphorus	0·100	Vitamin B_{12}	0·0003		
Magnesium	0·010				

atoms. The fatty acids commonly found in other foods – meat fat, olive oil, maize oil and the like – possess molecules containing sixteen and eighteen carbon atoms.

The source of the lower fatty acids in the milk of ruminants was for a long time a mystery. Then in the 1950s it was discovered that they were formed from acetic acid, CH_3. COOH, which is produced when the micro-organisms in the cow's rumen break down the carbohydrate they derive from the straw and husk and other fibrous materials which they eat. The discovery was made in two stages. First it was found that the main end-product of carbohydrate fermentation in a cow's rumen is acetic acid. Then by making acetic acid containing so-called 'labelled' ^{14}C carbon atoms in its molecules in place of some of the ^{12}C of which normal acetic acid is composed and giving this to lactating cows, it was possible to trace what was happening to the acetic acid. By this means it was found that all the 'lower fatty acids', that is the peculiarly 'buttery' C_4-fatty acid, butyric acid, became 'labelled'. It was therefore deduced that acetic acid and the fatty acid derived from it originate in the rumen. Higher fatty acids containing 18 carbon atoms or more did not contain significant amounts of the 'labelled' carbon.

Several practical implications arise from this kind of knowledge. The first is perhaps a trivial one: it is that cow's milk and butter possess the taste and consistency they do to a marked degree because the cow is a ruminating animal. Secondly it has already

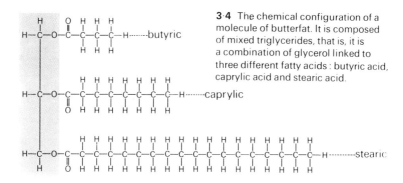

3·4 The chemical configuration of a molecule of butterfat. It is composed of mixed triglycerides, that is, it is a combination of glycerol linked to three different fatty acids : butyric acid, caprylic acid and stearic acid.

glycerol

been shown that the amount of acetic acid a cow obtains, either by being given it direct or as a component of fermented silage, or from the fermentation of roughage in its own rumen, is increased not only in the butter-fat content of its milk, but also in the total amount of milk produced. It thus appears that understanding the activity of endocrine hormones is only one way in which the quality and quantity of milk secretion may be controlled. Understanding the cows dietary needs and metabolic processes offers an alternative method of control, but in this rather subtle way.

Feeding in general terms exerts an influence more on the quantity of milk than on its quality. Certain feed components, notably vitamin A and carotene (a pigment derived from green pasture plants which contributes to vitamin A-activity) do, however, directly affect milk composition. Summer milk from cows grazing in the fields contains more vitamin A-activity than milk from stall-fed cows. The genetical background of the cow has a significant influence on the composition of its milk. This not only implies that certain individual cows yield milk that is higher in fat or protein than others. It also follows that particular breeds of cattle give milk with a characteristic composition. The so-called Channel Island breeds, Jerseys and Guernseys, produce milk with a high fat content. On the other hand, some strains of Friesian or Holstein breed can be developed to yield very large volumes of milk in which the concentration not only of fat but also of protein is reduced so far below what is expected from cows' milk that it can almost be argued that the marketing of such milk by commercial producers amounts to 'biological adulteration'.

But although the breeding of milk cattle for excessive yield accompanied by poor nutritional quality may lead to undesirable consequences, the application of scientific methods to the breeding of high-yielding cows and the improved understanding of the nutritional requirements of dairy cattle have led to a continuous improvement in the productivity of cows considered as biological machines for the manufacture of milk for human consumption. For example, in the decade 1935 to 1945 the average annual production of milk per cow rose from 4,180 – 4,800 lb a year, an increase of 15%.

The food value of milk The figures which have already been given in table 2·2 and in table 3·3 imply that milk provides protein of good nutritional quality – fat, vitamin A-activity, the B-vitamins, thiamine, riboflavin, niacin, pantothenic acid, inositol and vitamin B_{12}, as well as numerous mineral elements. Since the milk of female mammals is intended as the sole food for the early days of their offspring, it can be expected that the process of evolution has brought the composition of such milk to suit exactly the nutritional needs of the young of that species. To fit cow's milk to the needs of human infants, as reference to table 3·1 shows, its protein concentration needs to be reduced. Otherwise it is well adapted to the early days of a child's nutrition. Milk, however, is – at least in the wealthier industrial countries – fed to other than infants. It is given to children and adolescents and also to adults. For people it has certain valuable attributes. As a liquid, it is a remarkably concentrated vehicle for nutrients. Furthermore, it is easy to consume. A pint, or half a litre, can be readily consumed at a draught. An equal weight of few other foods can be taken so conveniently and absorbed so readily.

But although the food value of milk is high and it contributes a broad spectrum of diverse nutrients it is not, as is sometimes claimed, a 'perfect' food for other than infants and, even for them, is so only for a comparatively limited period of their early life.

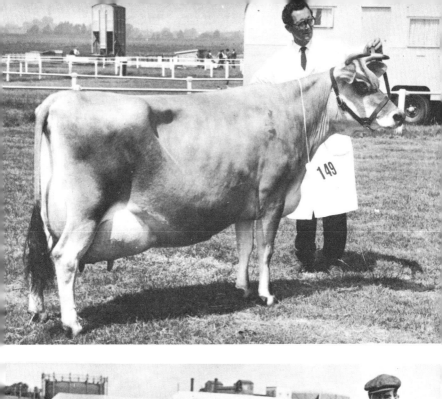
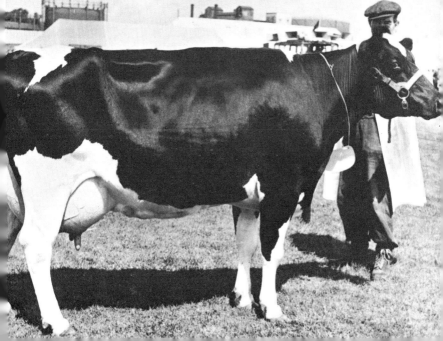

52

Table 3·4 Nutrients in whole raw milk

Protein	3·4%	Riboflavin	150 µg/100 g
Fat	3·6%	Pantothenic acid	300 µg/100 g
Carbohydrate	4·8%	Nicotinic acid	80 µg/100 g
Calcium	0·12%	Vitamin B_6	25 µg/100 g
Vitamin A	150 iu/100 g	Biotin	1·5 µg/100 g
Vitamin D	2 iu/100 g	Vitamin B_{12}	0·3 µg/100 g
Thiamine	45 µg/100 g	Vitamin C	2·0 µg/100 g

Milk contains only the merest trace of iron. The liver of an infant born by a well-nourished mother contains a store of iron amply sufficient for its first stage of life and milk is, therefore, 'perfectly' adapted to the needs of such an infant. But when it constitutes a major proportion of the diet of any individual other than an infant, its lack of iron seriously detracts from its nutritional completeness. In fact, this lack of iron in milk makes it popular with scientists researching in nutrition as a specifically iron-free anaemia-producing diet for experimental animals. The second shortcoming of milk arises from the chemical reactivity of vitamin C.

The molecular structure of vitamin C (ascorbic acid) is such that it can readily become oxidised. Indeed, this oxidisability is an integral part of its biochemical function. There is enough vitamin C in milk sucked by an infant directly from its mother to supply its nutritional needs. When, however, milk is collected as a commodity for distribution through the channels of commerce as a foodstuff for general use, the limited amount of vitamin C in it can readily be lost. The riboflavin also present in milk acts, particularly in the presence of light, as a catalyst to bring about the oxidation of vitamin C. It follows, therefore, that an all-milk diet can easily be deficient in vitamin C.

Cheese

At the beginning of the present century, cows were kept at the outskirts of cities or actually within the towns themselves. This happened because milk, although it is a useful and nutritious food, is highly susceptible to infection. In other words, milk is perishable and quickly 'goes bad' unless special steps are taken to prevent it doing so. Even when industrialisation developed and transport facilities improved with the advent of railways for the delivery of milk from the country into the towns, it was impossible to avoid considerable wastage by souring during the summer months. Because of this, many farmers sold milk to the towns only during the winter and during the summer months they converted the main substance of their cow's milk into the more stable foodstuff, cheese.

On farms situated at a still greater distance from the centres of population in the towns where the main market for liquid milk was to be found, cheese-making was perforce the main product where the soil and climate were nevertheless suitable for dairying. In Great Britain, the most important of such areas were the south-west of Scotland, where Dunlop cheese was made; the Cheshire region, including considerable areas of North Wales, Staffordshire and Shropshire, as well as Cheshire itself – where Cheshire cheese was made; the Somerset area, which was the original home of Cheddar cheese, and the north Midlands with Derby and Stilton cheese. Similar considerations applied to other European countries and, later on, the areas of North America suited to milk producing but situated even further from any market naturally became centres for the development of cheese production, often combined with the raising of pigs which could be fed on the whey left over as a by-product of the cheese manufacture.

Cheese is a convenient medium for concentrating the main nutrients of milk, the protein and fat, the calcium, vitamin A and part of the milk sugar, lactose.

Cheese-making goes back to remotest antiquity. The Bible contains a number of references to it. For example, in the second book

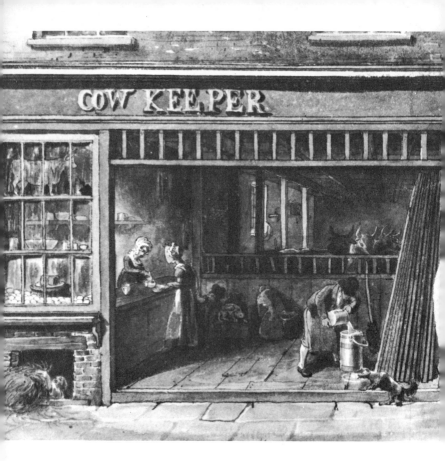

of Samuel there is the report that 'when David was come to Mahanaim, that Shobi the son of Nahash ... and Machir the son of Ammiel of Lo-debar and Barzillai the Gilliadite ... brought beds and basins and earthen vessels and wheat and barley and flour and parched corn and beans and lentiles and parched pulse and honey and butter and sheep and cheese of kine [that is, cheese made from cow's milk] – ... for they said, The people is hungry and weary and thirsty in the wilderness.' (II Samuel 17, 27–29). It will be noted that this list, including cheese, comprises foods all of which are comparatively non-perishable. Then again in the Book of Job, chapter 10, there is the even more illuminating passage

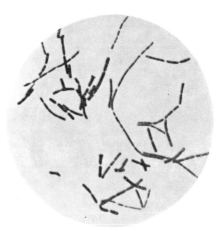

3·6 Left Seventy years ago cows were kept within or on the outskirts of towns because there was no way of preventing milk from souring or of transporting it quickly from country areas. **Right** Photomicrograph of *Lactobacillus acidophilus*. The bacteria produce acid in milk during the process of cheese-making. **Below** Cheese-making in Britain in the 18th century.

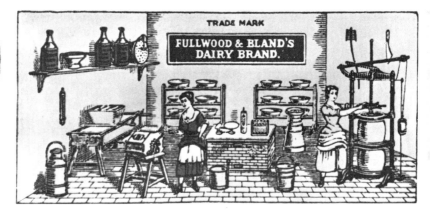

TRADE MARK

FULLWOOD & BLAND'S DAIRY BRAND.

(*v.* 10) in which the prophet, referring to the state to which his misfortunes have reduced him, exclaims, 'Hast thou not poured me out as milk, and curdled me like cheese?' This clearly refers to the action of the enzyme rennin, which is the active component of the preparation rennet, made from calves' stomachs which is used, even in the present technological processes for coagulating the protein of milk and thus allowing it, and the various other components to which I have referred, to be separated from much of the water, which is the major constituent of liquid milk.

Besides the people of the Old Testament, the Greeks and Romans also appear to have used cheese as a staple food at least a thousand years before the beginning of the Christian era. Its nutritional significance was recognised as well as its convenience as a food which could be carried on the march without deteriorating, for both the Jews and the Romans used it as a military ration. The Greeks included it in the diet given to wrestlers to increase their endurance.

Although cheese does not contain all the nutrients of the milk from which it is made, since a proportion of the B-vitamins and a proportion of the sugar which is converted into lactic acid are removed with the whey, it can in general be taken that the main

Table 3·5 Nutrients in Cheddar cheese

Protein	26·0%	Pantothenic acid	2–4 μg/g
Fat	33·0%	Vitamin B_6	0·2–0·5 μg/g
Calcium	0·7–1·1%	Biotin	0·01—0·03 μg/g
Vitamin A	8–16 iu/g	Vitamin B_{12}	0·01–0·03 μg/g
Thiamine	0·3–0·6 μg/g	Nicotinic acid	0·3–1·2 μg/g
Riboflavin	3–7 μg/g		

Table 3·6 Composition of cheeses (per 100 g)

	Water	Kilo-calories	Protein	Fat	Carbo-hydrate
	g		g	g	g
Camembert	52·2	299	17·5	24·7	1·8
Cheddar	37·0	398	25·0	32·2	2·1
Limburger	45·0	345	21·2	28·0	2·2
Parmesan	30·0	393	36·0	26·0	2·9
Roquefort	40·0	368	21·5	30·5	2·0

nutrients from 100 lb of milk are concentrated into 8 to 13 lb of cheese, depending on the method of preparation. Over the centuries, cheeses of many sorts, textures and flavours have been made throughout the world. In principle, the process by which cheese is prepared from milk involves first of all acidity. Bacteria which produce lactic acid, so called *lactobacilli*, are widespread throughout the terrestrial environment. Simple souring of milk causes curdling. The separated 'curds' are, indeed, sometimes called soft cheese. Harder varieties of cheese are, as was implied by the Book of Samuel, prepared by the use of the enzyme rennin.

A molecule of casein, or of other proteins in milk, possesses a complex spatial configuration. The enzyme rennin changes this molecular shape in a way, the details of which have yet to be fully understood. The effect of this molecular change is, however, to prevent the newly shaped molecule fitting into the 'mesh' of water molecules. Hence, the protein comes out of solution. The clot so formed entangles the fat and many of the other components of the milk. By being cut and worked mechanically, and by the action of diverse other bacteria and moulds which inhabit the varied environments in which different cheeses have traditionally been made, the amount of water retained by the cheese, the proportion of fat enmeshed and a host of trace components contributing to

Calcium	Iron	Vitamin A	Thiamine	Ribo-flavin	Niacin	Vitamin C
mg	mg	iu	mg	mg	mg	mg
105	0·5	1,010	0·04	0·75	0·80	0
750	1·0	1,300	0·03	0·46	0·10	0
590	0·6	1,140	0·08	0·50	0·20	0
1,140	0·4	1,060	0·02	0·73	0·20	0
315	0·5	1,240	0·03	0·61	1·20	0

smell and colour and taste – all these are affected and so lead to the final idiosyncratic composition and character of the final cheese.

The composition of a number of cheeses is shown in table 3·6.

Other concentrated milk fractions

Cheese represents the most complete concentrate of the nutrients from milk. Everything is in it except part of the mineral elements and some of the B-vitamins. Indeed, cheese is remarkable for its antiquity, its completeness as a foodstuff, for its diverse character reflecting the variability of the bacterial flora used to bring about the production of lactic acid by which the souring is accomplished and by its durability as a food capable of resisting storage. There are, however, other commodities in which concentration of milk components has been accomplished, if to a less complete degree. The simplest is the separation of *cream*. The butter fat in milk, present as a suspension of globules, has a natural tendency to rise. It can then be removed by skimming or by being spun away from the milk in a mechanical centrifuge.

Cream contains almost all the fat and usually one third to half of the protein and lactose of the milk from which it is separated. It consequently contains much of the vitamin A content of the milk but lacks the protein and the calcium. Clotted cream, also called Devonshire cream, is made by separating the fat by a process of heating in special pans. But the commonest preparation of milk fat is butter. Cream is an emulsion in which fat globules are suspended in an aqueous solution. The mechanical action of churning causes an 'inversion' of the emulsion; butter is therefore a suspension of aqueous globules in a fat. In India, the process is taken further. Butter is heated so that the aqueous globules settle out and the clarified fat can then be separated as *ghee*. Because the watery part has been removed, there is less opportunity for bacterial action so that the ghee keeps well in the warm climate.

There are less complete concentrates to be found in a number of countries. In the West, so-called cream cheese, or cottage cheese,

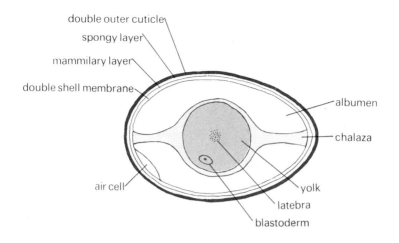

contains more water and less fat than normal cheeses. Yoghurt is a sour milk preparation originally made in Greece, Rumania, Hungary, Bulgaria, Turkey and parts of the Soviet Union from the milk of cows, goats, sheep or buffaloes; kefir is a similar product made in the Caucasus; kumiss is a drink made from mares' milk in Russia and dahi is a sour milk preparation widely used in India.

Eggs and the manufacturing capabilities of the hen

Milk is the fluid excreted by a mammal for the nourishment of its newly independent foetus until the foetus becomes capable of utilising for itself the foodstuffs that the general environment supplies. We make use of this ability of mammals, such as the cow, the water-buffalo, the mare, the goat and the sheep to manufacture palatable, concentrated and culinarily convenient foods – and drink their milk. Birds and reptiles do not suckle their young. They start them in life, as a fertilised embryo, in a closed container – an egg. But, like mammals, they provide them with a supply of concentrated, nutritionally well-balanced foods to sustain them throughout the early period of their development when they are unable to pick up a living for themselves. And we treat hens – and ducks, seagulls, plovers, pigeons and geese – like cows, and eat their eggs.

The efficiency of a modern hen, scientifically bred for egg-laying, as a physiological machine for manufacturing human food for man,

3·8 The original Jungle Fowl (*below*), from which modern fowls have been bred, lays only 20–25 eggs a year. The Light Sussex Hen (*right*) lays between 140 and 175 eggs a year when kept on free-range. Modern battery hens lay from 250–300 eggs annually, making them second only to the cow as food producers.

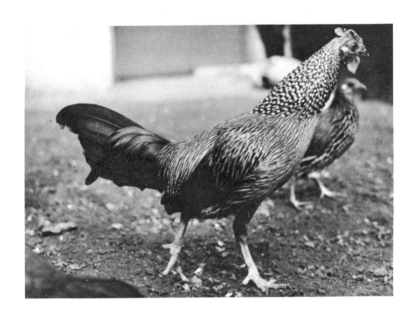

Table 3·7 Composition of eggs (per 100 g)

	Water	Kilo-calories	Protein	Fat	Carbo-hydrate
	g		g	g	g
Hen's egg	73·7	163	12·9	11·5	0·9
Duck's egg	70·4	191	13·3	14·5	0·7
Goose's egg	70·4	185	13·9	13·3	1·3
Turkey's egg	72·6	170	13·1	11·8	1·7

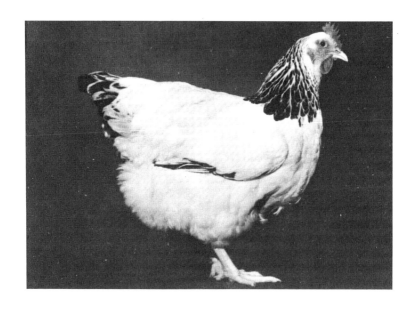

Calcium	Iron	Vitamin A	Thiamine	Ribo- flavin	Niacin	Vitamin C
mg	mg	iu	mg	mg	mg	mg
54	2·3	1,180	0·30	0·30	0·1	0
56	2·8	1,230	0·18	0·30	0·1	0
—	—	—	—	—	—	—
—	—	—	—	—	—	—

is phenomenal. The original jungle fowl from which the sophisticated poultry of today are descended laid only 20 to 25 eggs a year. Today, hens lay 300 eggs a year and those capable of 250 are common. This means that selective breeding has created a highly specialised biological machine for the conversion of raw materials into human food. A 2-kilo hen laying 250 eggs is manufacturing and packing 15 kilos of finished product each year. This performance is second only to that of an 'improved' cow.

Since the white, which is mainly protein, and the yolk of egg, which is rich in fat, must provide the entire subsistence for a bird, which is a creature of quite high biological complexity, it is hardly surprising that the two together constitute a food of excellent dietary value for man. The composition of hens' eggs is shown in table 3·7. It can be seen to contain almost every nutrient except vitamin C. The protein contains the so-called 'essential' amino acids in proportions well suited to the nutrition of human children and adults as was implied in table 2·2. The fat contains vitamins A and D, whereas milk lacks iron; iron is present in comparatively high proportion in egg yolk. But to illustrate once again that, no matter how valuable a commodity may be as a component of a mixed diet, no one article can be claimed as a perfect food by itself, egg contains cholesterol of which too much in the diet can be harmful; it also contains, when raw, a curious compound called *avidin* capable of immobilising the vitamin biotin and thus inducing vitamin deficiency.

4 Cereals, vegetables and fruits

Cereals

When the New Testament says, 'for all flesh is as grass, and all the glory of man as the flower of grass,' the words have truth both in a spiritual and in a material sense. All the cereals which have provided the basis upon which the civilisations of the world have been developed – rice, wheat, rye, barley, oats and maize, sorghum and millet – all these are, botanically, members of the grass family. Only when ancient man had discovered that these plants could be cultivated to provide a source of food which was easy to grow and which could be preserved from one season to the next was it possible for roving bands to be transformed into settled communities. And because the growing of cereals required much less of men's time than the laborious and uncertain pursuit of wild animals and fish, they began to have time to spare for the arts and sciences of civilisation.

Of all the cereals, wheat is most widely used. It will grow under a wide variety of conditions although the best wheat-growing areas are in the temperate zones where the rainfall is from 13 to 35 inches a year. Barley, oats and rye are adapted to much the same conditions, but most communities prefer wheat, the flour of which, containing the protein gluten, is particularly well suited to the making of bread. Rye, however, can survive more severe winters than wheat and is, in consequence, sown in some northern countries. It also thrives remarkably well on soils of low fertility.

Rice is extensively grown in warmer, humid parts of the world and forms the staple food for a substantial proportion of the human race. Maize was originally indigenous to North America but was brought to Europe by Christopher Columbus, since which time it has become a major crop in the Danube basin and elsewhere.

Although the various cereals differ from each other in a number of respects, they demonstrate their common ancestry by a general similarity in food value. They all provide calories by virtue of the starch in their endosperm. But, at the same time, they are all deficient in calcium and vitamin A – except yellow maize – and the biological value (that is, the relative amounts of amino acids) of their protein is less satisfactory than that of the proteins found in animal foods. None of them, when used, as they are, as dried seeds, contains any vitamin C.

Cereals were eaten as a form of porridge long before bread was invented and porridge was succeeded by flat unleavened cakes. It is interesting to note that even today certain African communities still continue to consume their cereals as porridge or gruel, while Scottish oatcake, Indian chappaties and Jewish matzos represent the early pre-bread forms of cereal preparation. Finally, the production of the wheaten loaf, a sign of cultural development, was attained successively by the Egyptians, the Greeks and then the Romans.

Although both wheat and barley were certainly in use in the late bronze age, wheat gradually displaced barley as the main food for man, barley being mainly given to domestic animals. And comparatively early in history, the people using wheat began to 'improve' it by what amounted to a process of selective breeding, just as had been done for cattle and poultry. By the end of the classical period, so-called naked wheats, more suitable for bread-making, had been distinguished from the *emmer* or hulled wheats. These had been difficult to dehusk; in fact, the 'threshing' process for emmer wheat had probably consisted of burning off the ears, thus giving rise to the 'parched corn' of the Bible. A further example of the advantage to be gained from guided plant breeding was recognition by both the Greeks and the Romans of the technical characteristics of 'hard' wheat (*Triticum*) and 'soft' wheat (*Siligo*) with different milling and baking properties. In fact, 'hard' wheat contains protein, the chemical configuration of which enables it to be drawn out into the strong, fine, elastic structure of a firm yet 'light' loaf, whereas the protein in 'soft' wheat pulls out into more fragile, less elastic dough which, while less suited to bread-making, makes it a better biscuit flour. Both proteins are of substantially the same chemical composition, it is the three-dimensional geometry of the molecules that is different.

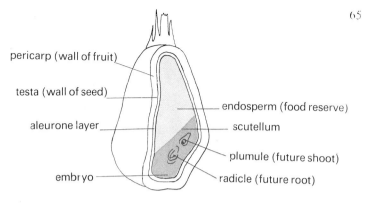

pericarp (wall of fruit)

testa (wall of seed)

endosperm (food reserve)

aleurone layer

scutellum

plumule (future shoot)

embryo

radicle (future root)

The invention of mills for grinding 'corn' goes back to remote antiquity and from very early times steps were taken to free flour from at least a proportion of the husk of the grain. The practice of sieving and 'bolting' grist was carried out in many different parts of the world by as early as AD 50. It has been estimated that at the time of Pliny, about 50 per cent of the total grain was separated as best-quality white flour when soft wheats were used and 30 per cent from hard wheat. When only standard quality bread-baking flour was required, about 85 per cent of the grist from either wheat was used. It is interesting to find that Galen graded the four kinds of flour that were in use in his time (second century AD) from the point of view of their nutritional value. He rated 'best white' as having the highest nutritional value, 'seconds' came next, then 'wholemeal', and he placed 'bran bread', which was made largely from millers' offals and eaten by the poorest people, as least nutritious of all. He also noticed that the 'bran bread' produced the largest bulk of faeces and the 'best white' the least. These conclusions can in the main be supported by current scientific opinion.

There have been two major scientific and technological developments in the use of wheat which have radically affected the food supplies of at least the western half of the world during the last hundred years or so. The first was the introduction of silk bolting cloths for sifting out the fine white flour together with, in about 1870, the replacement of mill-stones, which in one form or another had been in use for thousands of years, by steel rollers. The second major innovation was the application of the science of genetics to the breeding of new strains of wheat.

The silk bolting cloths and steel mills were first introduced into

4·2 Wheat passing through rolling mills. The rollers crack open the grain without powdering it. Rolling and subsequent sieving separate the husk and embryo from the rest of the grain, producing white flour with little fat, which would quickly turn it rancid.

Hungary and the United States to cope with the 'hard' wheats grown in those countries. The importation of hard American wheats into Europe in due course led to the general use of steel rollers in milling plants in all countries in which the nineteenth-century technology was developing. The significance of the steel rollers in milling lay in the fact that stone grinding pounded up the grain so that, no matter how meticulously the subsequent sifting was done, it was impossible completely to separate the last traces of husk and embryo from the flour. When steel rollers were introduced, however, a pair of initial rolls could be arranged to crack open the grain without fragmenting it into powder, followed by a sieve to separate the 'offal' from the 'semolina'. Then the 'offal' was put through a second pair of smooth rollers. These flattened the embryo, enabling it to be picked up by a second sieve set underneath the rollers. Thus, by passing the flour streams through a sequence of 'break' rolls and 'reduction' rolls it was possible to produce white flour entirely free from the husk and the other layers of the grain and, more particularly, from the embryo.

Table 4·1 Composition of wheat and flour (per 100 g)

	Kilocalories	Protein
		g
Wheat	328	13·6
endosperm (85%)		8·5
bran and aleurone (12%)		9·0
scutellum (1·5%)		24·3
embryo (1·0%)		30·4
Flour		
85% extraction	339	13·6
80% extraction	341	13·2
70% extraction	341	12·8

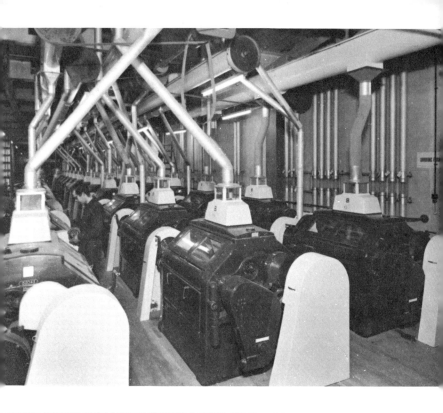

Fat	Fibre	Thiamine	Riboflavin	Niacin
g	g	mg	mg	mg
2·5	2·2	0·37	0·12	3·5
1·1	—	0·48	0·07	2·2
4·1	10·8	0·45	0·50	25·0
30·3	—	16·55	1·50	6·0
15·4	2·5	0·90	1·50	6·0
1·7	0·3	0·29	0·07	2·1
1·4	0·1	0·24	0·06	1·6
1·2	trace	0·08	0·05	1·2

Because the embryo contains a comparatively high proportion of fat, flour in which traces of it are present becomes rancid if it is stored for any length of time.

In early days, white flour and white bread made from it were highly prized by the richest people. Indeed, Antiphanes, before 350 BC, wrote about 'lovely white loaves filling the oven'. After the introduction of modern milling equipment, white bread, free of embryo and with good keeping qualities, became cheaper than brown bread which, in consequence, acquired a certain prestige among the well-to-do. Table 4·1 shows the chemical composition of different parts of the wheat grain and of flours milled in different ways.

The figures given in table 4·1 show up a number of points. First of all it can be seen that the embryo and the scutellum – the 'shield' which separates it from the endosperm where the starch is stored in the seed – contain a disproportionately large amount of fat. This is why flour milled in modern equipment, particularly to an 'extraction rate' of 70 per cent or even less, keeps better than flour in which a significant amount of embryo has been allowed to remain. On the other hand it can be seen that the scutellum, a structure constituting only 1 per cent of the total weight of the wheat grain, contains 200 times the concentration of thiamine present in white 70 per cent-extraction flour. These facts have a bearing on whether brown bread, made from flour of a high extraction rate, is more nourishing than white bread. This is a less straightforward question than it seems. Indeed, it cannot reasonably be discussed in the context simply of cereal chemistry but relates to the total problem of industrialised society as a whole. I shall, therefore, defer discussing it until chapter 8.

If one modern development in the use of cereals, and particularly wheat, for food has been this innovation in its preparation as flour and bread, the second has been the application of biological science to increase the amount of wheat produced. The great expansion in food production during the past century has been only partly due to the discoveries in chemistry which have attracted most attention: the

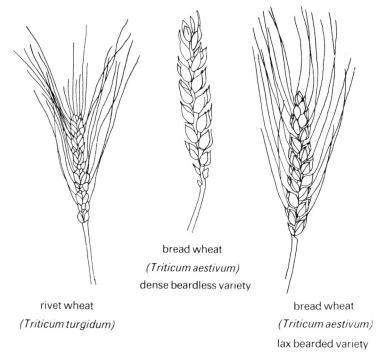

rivet wheat
(Triticum turgidum)

bread wheat
(Triticum aestivum)
dense beardless variety

bread wheat
(Triticum aestivum)
lax bearded variety

invention of chemical fertilisers, insecticides, fungicides and weed-killers. These have done much, but of far more significance has been the development by plant breeders and geneticists of the new varieties of wheat – Red Fife in the 1840s, then Marquis, then in the 1920s Ceres, followed by Thatcher, later succeeded by Regent. It was Red Fife and Marquis that enabled wheat to be grown for the first time over enormous areas of Canada further north and west than ever before, where the season was too short and the rainfall too sparse to allow the then existing varieties to thrive. But wheat is not only subject to drought and frost. Like man, each of the cereal crops is subject to destructive diseases. In 1916, when Alberta was sown with Marquis, there came an epidemic of the fungus disease, 'stem rust'. It was estimated that in one year alone 100 million bushels of wheat were lost.

No preventive treatment was known, no cure could be found. Chemical dips and sprays were unavailing. The solution to the problem lay with the cereal breeders who succeeded in producing,

4·4 Loose smut of wheat. Breeding has produced strains of wheat resistant to attack by this fungus, thereby greatly increasing productivity.

one after another, the strains which I have named. It can thus be seen that, just as has been done with beef cattle, sheep and pigs, the cereal breeders have mated selected stock to get an 'improved' wheat. But more than this, they have bred varieties not only to yield increased amounts of food but also to resist disease – that is, to cope with the ecological stresses of their environment. When the meat producers become dissatisfied with the few strains of Short-horn, Friesian, Jersey and Charrolais cattle and start seriously cropping wild ungulates for the market they will have reached the point at which cereal breeders are now. As with wheat, similar progress has been made in breeding rice, maize and other crops.

The cereals, as can be seen from table 4·2, contribute variable amounts of protein, although this protein is somewhat deficient in the amino acid lysine, and many also contain useful amounts of the B-vitamins, depending on the way in which they have been milled. There is a peculiarity about maize. Where maize constituted a major part of the diet, as it did at one time in some parts of the United States and in Egypt, the disease, pellagra, was endemic. Pellagra occurs when people obtain insufficient of the vitamin

Table 4·2 Composition of the more important cereal grains (per 100 g)

	Kilocalories	Protein	Fat	Calcium
		g	g	mg
Wheat	340	12	2	38
Rice (brown)	310	8	2	32
Maize (yellow)	352	10	4	22
Sorghum	348	10	4	28
Oats	317	10	5	60
Rye	338	11	2	50

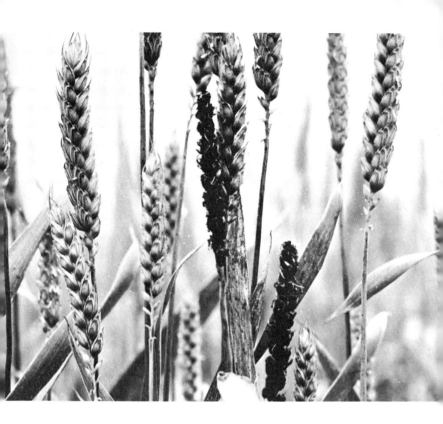

Iron	Vitamin A	Thiamine	Riboflavin	Niacin
mg	iu	mg	mg	mg
3·1	0	0·57	0·12	4·3
1·6	0	0·34	0·05	4·7
2·1	490	0·37	0·12	2·2
4·4	0	0·38	0·15	3·9
3·8	0	0·50	0·14	1·3
3·5	0	0·27	0·10	1·2

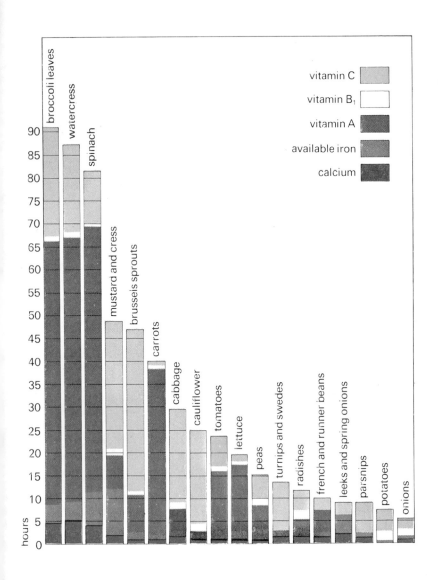

4.5 The chart shows how many hours supply of various nutrients there are in 4 oz portions of different vegetables.

Legend:
- vitamin C
- vitamin B₁
- vitamin A
- available iron
- calcium

Vegetables (left to right): broccoli leaves, watercress, spinach, mustard and cress, brusseis sprouts, carrots, cabbage, cauliflower, tomatoes, lettuce, peas, turnips and swedes, radishes, french and runner beans, leeks and spring onions, parsnips, potatoes, onions

y-axis: hours (0, 5, 10, 15, 20, 25, 30, 35, 40, 45, 50, 55, 60, 65, 70, 75, 80, 85, 90) niacin in their diet. Maize, however, does not contain strikingly less niacin than some other cereals. It was later discovered, however, that the protein of maize was not only lacking in lysine but also contained very little of a second amino acid, tryptophan, which exerts an effect, less pronounced than niacin but nevertheless significant, in preventing pellagra.

Vegetables

If for the moment we exclude potatoes, what are generally called 'vegetables' are, with the exception of dried peas and beans, negligible sources of calories. In the form in which they are customarily eaten most vegetables are from 90 to 95 per cent water, that is to say, they contain more water than milk and about as much as beer. Their main significance in diet is as a source of vitamin C. In addition they contribute useful amounts of vitamin A-activity. The food value of vegetables is shown diagrammatically in figure 4·5. A curious feature about the use of vegetables as food, however, is not what we know about their composition but what we either do not know or never consider. For example, the major proportion of the dry matter of what we eat as 'vegetables' consists of carbohydrate. Part of this is made up of normal starch and sugars which are readily utilised as food. But part is composed of inulin which is broken down into fructose, unlike starch which yields glucose. In vegetables of the Compositae family, that is, Jerusalem artichokes, globe artichokes, chicory and salsify, between 30 and 40 per cent of the total carbohydrate is inulin. Although inulin and its breakdown products are absorbed into the body, their metabolism is different from that of starch. Pectins also follow an obscure metabolic pathway while galactans, which occur in peas and beans – and in seaweed – and hexosans such as lichenin and iso-lichenin, which are found notably in carrageen moss, are probably mainly utilised by way of the micro-flora of the gut. Indeed, their principal role in nutrition may well lie in the stimulating effect they produce on the glands of the digestive tract which

4·6 The chart shows how many hours supply of various nutrients there are in 4 oz portions of different fruits.

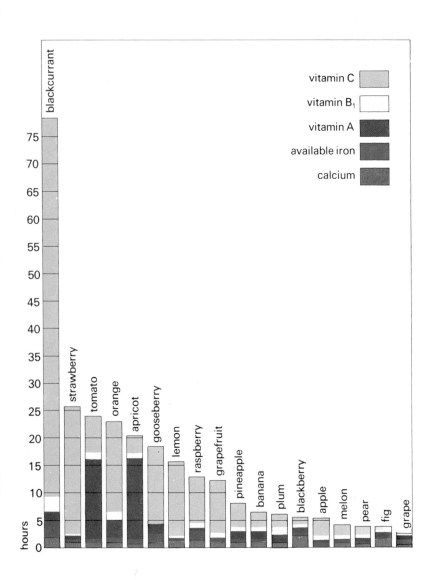

leads to an increase in the bulk of the faeces. In short, the chemical composition of many of the compounds in the dry matter of vegetables, commonly lumped together by analysts under the term, 'total carbohydrate', is not properly understood.

Although leaf vegetables only contain about 2 per cent of protein, it is worth pointing out – and this is often overlooked – that the dry matter of such vegetables contains more than twenty per cent of protein. A further point is that this protein is made up of a favourable proportion of constituent amino acids, particularly lysine which is present only in low concentration in cereal protein. Advantage is taken of the presence of this protein in leaves when they are specially processed to provide an extracted protein concentrate for populations whose diets are deficient in this nutrient. This is discussed in more detail in chapter 11.

Fruits

Fruits have been prized as lending variety and attractiveness to the diet since times of antiquity. Only when food science was beginning was doubt cast on their nutritional usefulness. This arose from the fact that from 75 to 90 per cent of their total weight is water. For the rest, about 1 per cent is protein and most fruits contain almost no fat. Only when it was discovered that fresh fruits contain vitamin C was their nutritional significance recognised. The relative food values of the main varieties of fruit are shown in figure 4·6.

Food technologists, as distinct from nutritionists, have from the first recognised that fruit is an agreeable article of diet much prized in every society and the variety of fruit available throughout the year to a modern civilised community is, more than any other type of foodstuff, almost entirely due to the application of scientific knowledge. For example, the banana was familiar to the armies of Alexander the Great when they were in India in 327 BC. Arab traders spread the growing of bananas across Africa to the Guinea coast from whence in 1482 the Portuguese took them to the Canary Islands. They were transported to the West Indies by the Spaniards in 1516 and from thence reached South America. But they were unknown in Europe, except as an exotic rarity, until about 1890 simply because no technical method was known of transporting them. It was only when it was discovered that they cannot tolerate a temperature below 13°C and ships and warehouses were carefully maintained above this value that the present very substantial world trade in bananas became possible.

The trade in oranges, too, grew only when plant geneticists had produced suitable varieties of trees and, above all, when means were found to protect each orange from the mould *Penicillium digitatum*, which otherwise causes them to rot in transit.

But the main discovery which today permits all sorts of fruit, apples, pears, South American plums, peaches as well as bananas, to be transported and stored and thus become available at almost any time of the year, was the recognition that all these are living entities. It follows, therefore, that the cells of an apple, let us say, maintain themselves alive, as we do, by the process of respiration. That is to say, they absorb oxygen and give off carbon dioxide. The process known as 'gas storage', by which apples can be kept in good condition throughout a long voyage halfway round the world followed by storage at a depot afterwards, involves the maintenance of a carefully controlled atmosphere containing regulated concentrations of carbon dioxide at a precisely adjusted temperature. By this means the life of the apples is prolonged.

Quite recently, food technologists and agriculturalists have been applying science to fruit in a new direction. As the standard of living in fruit-growing countries rises the cost of picking becomes an increasingly burdensome charge on the total cost of the fruit. To overcome this, the plant geneticists have developed varieties, for example, of raspberries capable of being picked by machinery. For example, there is a machine which has been developed by agricultural engineers to suit a modern cherry tree so that the cherries can be picked mechanically and their cost consequently reduced.

5 Oils and fats, sugars and spices

Oils and fats

The amount of fat in any particular diet is partly affected by the customs of the people whose food is being considered and is partly influenced by wealth. The diet of Eskimos contains a great deal of fat while that of the Kikuyu in East Africa contains very little. Under less extreme conditions, however, as communities become richer they tend to eat more fat. In 1900, the total amount of fat consumed by the British was 88 lb a head. This was made up of 82 per cent animal fat, 15 per cent vegetable fat, and 2 per cent from marine sources. By 1957, the fat consumption had increased to 113 lb a head, the proportion of animal fat had fallen to 69 per cent, the proportion of vegetable fat had increased to 26 per cent and that of marine fat to 6 per cent. But the 113 lb of fat consumed was not by any means made up solely of fats or oils in their recognisable forms. Less than half of the fat eaten was obtained as so-called 'visible' fat, the remainder was derived as integral com-

Table 5·1 Sources of fat in the British diet in 1957

Visible fat	Animal and vegetable fats and	lb/year
	oils eaten as such	20·0
	Butter	14·5
	Margarine	12·9
Invisible fat	Meat	37·6
	Milk, cheese	14·9
	Cereals and nuts	4·7
	Eggs	3·3
	Cocoa and chocolate	3·0
	Fish	1·9

5·1 Below The structure of cottonseed.
5·2 Right Coconuts being dried for making copra — the fibrous outer covering of the fruit. The coconut is a fruit having both nutritional and industrial uses.

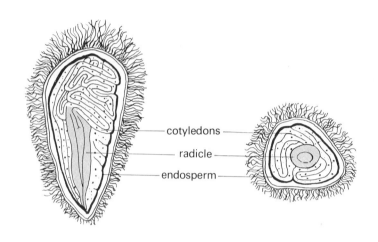

cotyledons

radicle

endosperm

ponents of other foods such as meat, milk and a variety of other articles. The main sources of fat in the food supplies of the United Kingdom are shown in table 5·1.

For the purposes of this chapter, I shall confine my discussion to the so-called cooking fats and oils and to margarine, that is to say to the 'visible' fats. The supply of these in industrialised countries is a matter of large-scale commerce and industry. The world has been combed for sources of fat; the developments of modern science make it immaterial what sort of fat or oil is available; any one sort can be refined, deodorised and, if necessary, hydrogenated so as to convert it into a useful, uniform article. The vegetable fats, comprising the main source of the total supply, are derived from cottonseed, a by-product, so to speak, of the cotton textile industry, from groundnuts, coconuts and soya beans. Other important sources are olives, sesame, palm and sunflower.

It is curious to observe that although cotton, which is an Indian plant, was known to the Greeks well before the Christian era and was extensively cultivated in the Mediterranean region at the time of the Mohammedan invasion in the seventh century, the use of

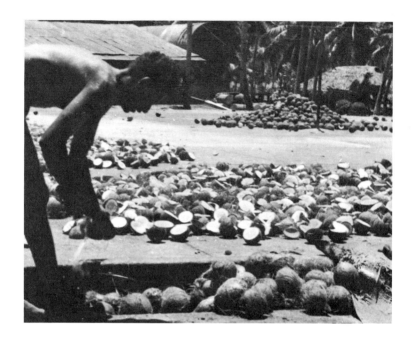

cottonseed as a source of fat for human consumption started only in the United States after the middle of the nineteenth century. The flower of the cotton plant is something like a single blossom off a hollyhock, to which it is in fact botanically related. By the time the pointed, blacky-brown seeds are mature they contain about 25 per cent of fat together with 30 per cent of protein.

While cottonseed oil is prepared as a major source of edible fat from a crop primarily grown for a quite different technical purpose, coconut oil – better described as coconut fat in view of the fact that it is solid at the normal atmospheric temperature of countries in the temperate parts of the world – is derived from a crop which is used as much for its technical as for its dietetic properties. Coconut, like cotton, has been of commercial significance for centuries. Its flesh is used directly for food as well as providing a source of oil, while the so-called coir fibre from its pericarp is utilised in making mats, matting, rope and cordage. At one time it was also extensively employed for caulking ships. The kernel contains about 37 per cent of fat and when dried in the traditional way in which it is handled as 'copra', 67 per cent of its substance is fat.

The two other main sources of edible vegetable oil in world commerce, soya beans and peanuts, both belong to the legume family and both have been known from remote antiquity. Soya beans have been cultivated in China and Japan since before written records were kept. Although they are grown today in many parts of the world, the main areas of production are still China, Japan and Korea, although large quantities are now grown in the United States. It is only during the last thirty years, however, that systematic plant breeding has been carried out to develop heavy cropping varieties giving high yields of oil. The amount of oil in properly cultivated soya beans exceeds 20 per cent.

Peanuts, which originally came from South America, grow at first in the way one would expect a legume to grow. The plants become about 2 ft high and have hairy stems. The pods grow about 2 in long and each contains up to 3 seeds. But after the flowers have withered, the stalks to which the pods are attached lengthen and bend over so that the seeds become forced underground where they ripen. Seeds of the large-seeded, large-podded varieties which have been bred for cultivation in the United States can contain up to 45 per cent of oil while other varieties with small pods and small seeds may yield 50 per cent or more.

It is important to realise that the current world trade in oils and fats, in which millions of tons of the diverse sorts are exported and imported is, in historical terms, a comparatively new phenomenon. Until the beginning of the present century, the only fats generally eaten were butter from the cow, beef suet from the ox and occasionally mutton suet from sheep and lard from the pig. 'Dripping' was often used in place of butter, and in Mediterranean countries, olive oil was used as well. The modern trade in fats is almost entirely a development of twentieth-century technology. It must also be remembered that this technology, besides leading to the use of fat extracted from soya beans, peanuts, coconuts and the like, also led to the release for human consumption of very large amounts of fat previously used for lamps.

Up till the latter end of the nineteenth century, artificial light was

5·3 Bottom part of the peanut plant – an important source of oil. The ends of the stems bearing the nuts eventually become subterranean and the nuts ripen underground.

almost entirely obtained from candles or from lamps fed with fatty oils which could otherwise have been eaten. The oil for lamps was, in Mediterranean countries, olive oil. In north-western Europe it was 'colza' or rape oil. Rape is a plant of the cabbage family (genus *Brassica*) and although its oil was never much prized for food, its seed contains up to 56 per cent of fat and the extracted residue was one of the first of such products to be employed as cattle cake. In the main, however, land was used to produce a potentially nutritious crop primarily for use, not as food, but as an illuminant. Even at the beginning of the present technological period of history rape oil was used in the lamps in railway carriages and in lighthouses.

Chemical composition of different fats Fats are, in chemical terms, a combination – a so-called ester – of the 3-carbon-atom alcohol, glycerol (sometimes called glycerine in common speech), and three fatty acids. The fatty acids are made up of chains of carbon atoms of various length terminated by a so-called *carboxyl* group which gives them their acid character. The consistency of a fat depends partly on the length of the carbon chain of its constituent fatty acids

Table 5·2 Saturated and unsaturated fatty acids and cholesterol in certain fats

	Saturated fatty acids	Unsaturated fatty acids	Cholesterol
	%	%	mg/100 g
Animal fats			
Lard	50	50	50
Beef tallow	55	45	75–140
Butter	48	52	240
Vegetable fats			
Coconut oil	90	10	Nil*
Palm oil	48	52	—
Cottonseed oil	25	75	—
Peanut oil	18	82	—
Olive oil	14	86	—
Soya bean oil	13	87	—

* Vegetable oils do not contain cholesterol but a substance of the same chemical class called phytosterol

and partly on whether the chain links are fully 'saturated' with hydrogen atoms. In general, the longer the chain, the higher is the melting point. It follows, therefore, that fats containing long-chain fatty acids tend to be solid at normal atmospheric temperature whereas fats made up of shorter chains may be expected to be liquids – that is to say, oils. But apart from chain length, the degree of saturation has a greater significance in two respects. First, of two fatty acids of the same number of carbon atoms, the more unsaturated one will possess the lower melting point – that is to say, it will be more liquid. The second significance of unsaturation is that it is associated with lower levels of cholesterol in the blood stream of people who eat the fat of which it is a part.

Cholesterol in one's blood stream has something to do with heart disease but, even after a decade of study, investigators are not sure what it does. The blood level of cholesterol is partly due to the amount of cholesterol eaten in food, partly due to the amount of 'saturated' fats and partly due to the amount of sugar in the diet.

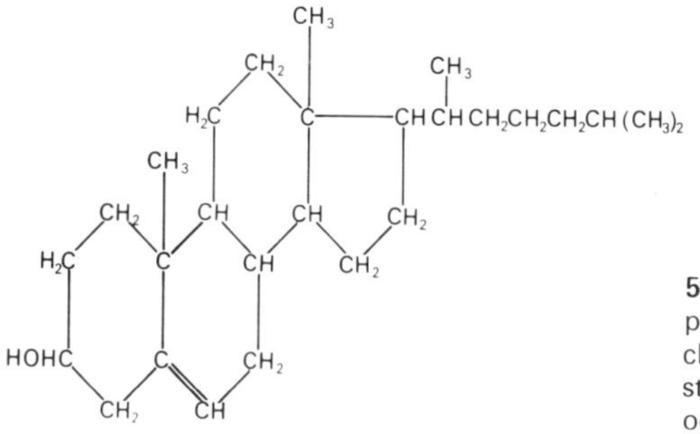

cholesterol

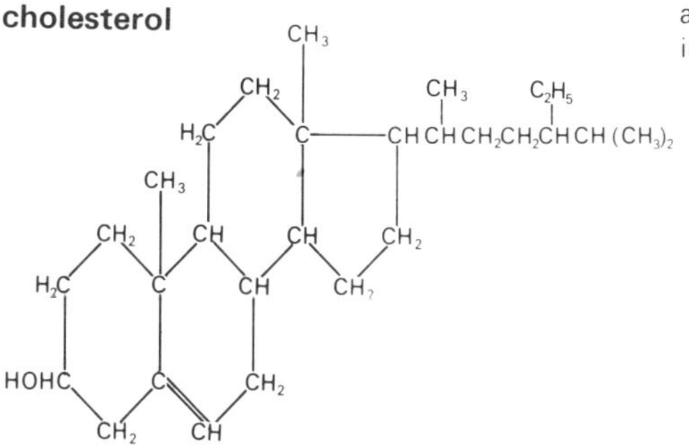

β sitosterol

5·4 Two compounds present in fats which are classified chemically as sterols. Cholesterol occurs in fats from animal sources; phytosterol in vegetable fats and oils.

All these cause the level to rise. On the other hand, certain 'unsaturated' fatty acids cause the level to fall and – most important of all – so does physical exercise. Here then is an only partly solved conundrum. And part of the key to the riddle may be in the facts set out in table 5·2.

Sugars

Just as compound cooking fat, margarine and the commerce in fats and oils from which they are manufactured are almost entirely a product of the modern age of science and technology, so also – though of somewhat older lineage – is sugar. During the last hundred years, the consumption of sugar in industrialised countries has increased sixfold. The amount consumed in Great Britain is now about 120 lb a year per head and the amount consumed in the United States exceeds 12 million tons a year. During the Middle Ages it was part of the spice trade that came from the East to

5·5 Today vast crops of sugar cane (*top*) are grown in tropical and subtropical areas, while sugar beet (*bottom*) is grown in temperate zones. New strains of plants and mechanical harvesting have made sugar, once a rarity, a common and widely used food. However, the large present-day consumption has several unfortunate effects on health.

Venice and thence into the rest of Europe. Even in the eighteenth century sugar was a luxury acquired from cane grown in tropical or semi-tropical areas of the Orient.

Today, vast areas of rich moist soil in many parts of the world are devoted to the production of sugar, from cane in the tropical and subtropical areas and from beet in temperate lands. Science has been brought to bear with enormous success on the breeding of more and more productive plants. It was only in 1858 that J.W. Parris, a planter in Barbados, first succeeded in growing to maturity sugar-cane seedlings and it was 1888 before such cultivation was recognised as a great new discovery. Since then a continuous increase in yield has been attained. And this is continuing. For example, the introduction of a newly-bred seed into Formosa in 1951 caused yields of sugar to rise 50 per cent by 1957. Similar continuous successes have been won over diseases and pests. Today the amount of sugar passing to and fro in international trade is little short of forty million tons a year, something less than two-thirds from cane and something more than one third from beet. Of this, about fifteen million tons is grown in North and Central America and the Caribbean, nine or ten million in Europe, four or five million tons in Asia and about four million tons in South America.

The strange thing is that this enormous trade in food has little to do with man's hunger and even less with his nutritional needs. Sugar, being pure carbohydrate, is a ready source of calories but, since it is solely carbohydrate, it contributes no protein, no minerals, no vitamins. Furthermore, it is one cause why teeth decay and it is incriminated in the coronary heart disease which afflicts the prosperous middle-aged men of the 'developed' countries. The enormous commerce in sugar, upon which whole communities depend for their economic support, has its main reason for existence in the fact that it is sweet. The significance of sweetness, its psychological and aesthetic basis, whether it contributes in any way to the physiological operations of the body or the survival of the race – all these are unknown.

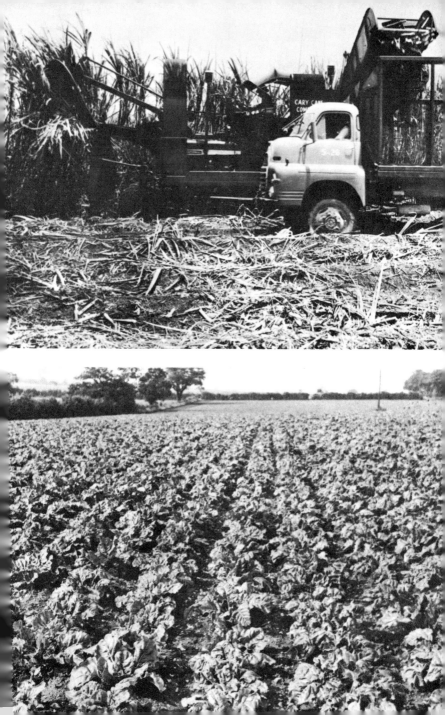

Table 5·3 Phenols and related constituents of volatile oils

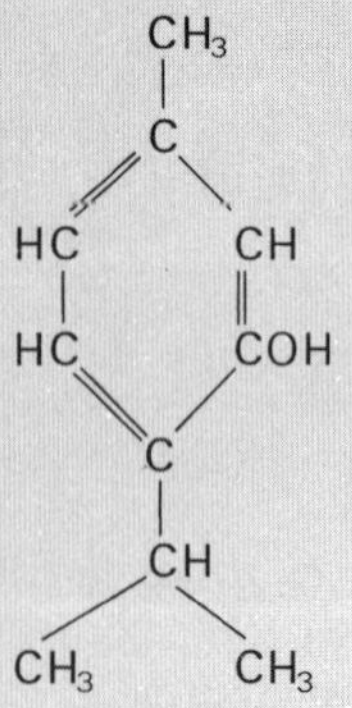

Thymol
(phenol)

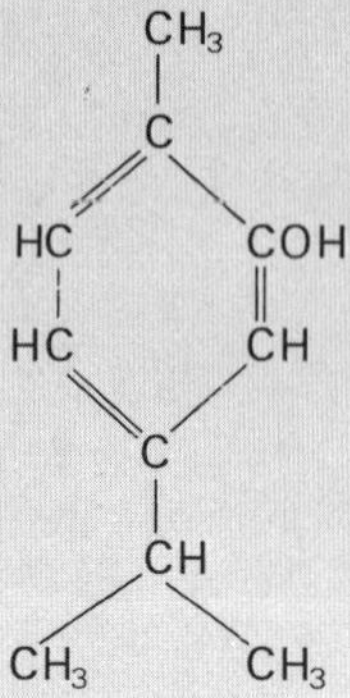

Carvacrol
(phenol)

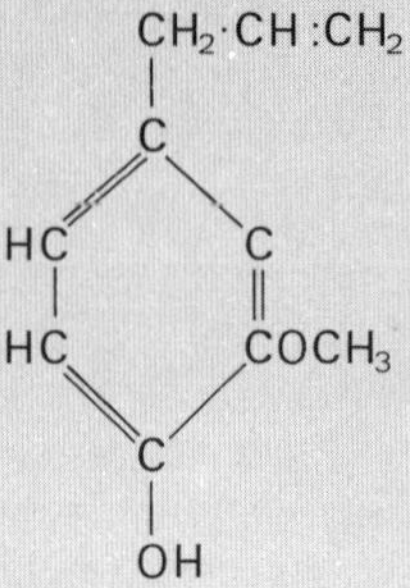

Eugenol
(phenol)

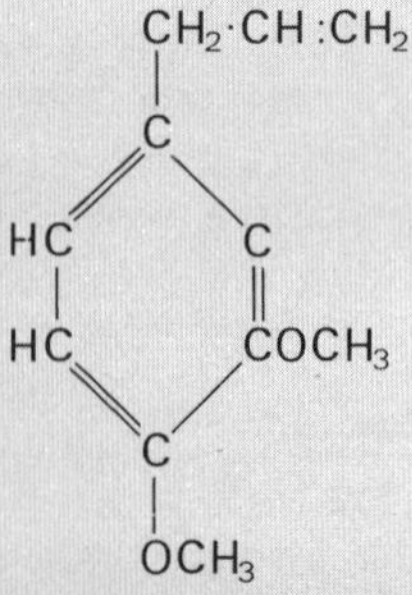

Methyl eugenol
(phenyl ester)

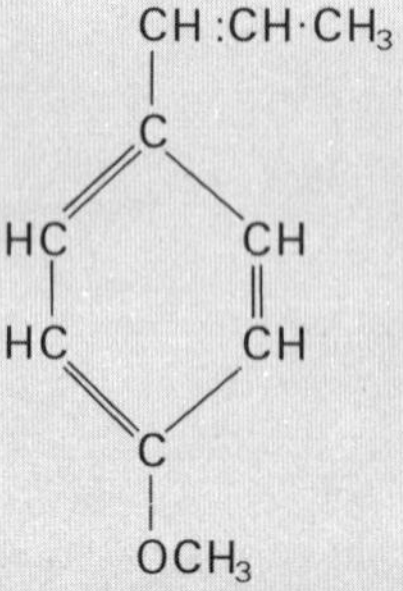

Anethole
(phenyl ester)

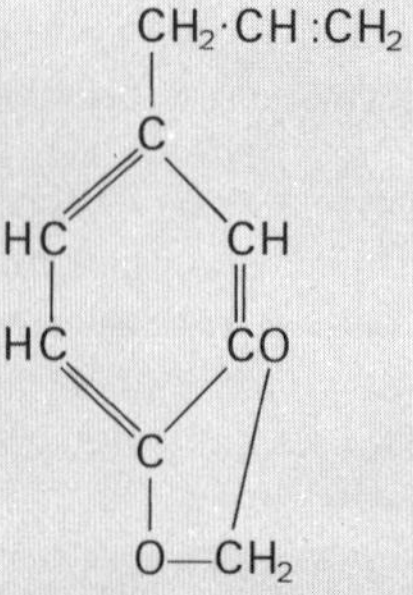

Safrole
(phenyl ester)

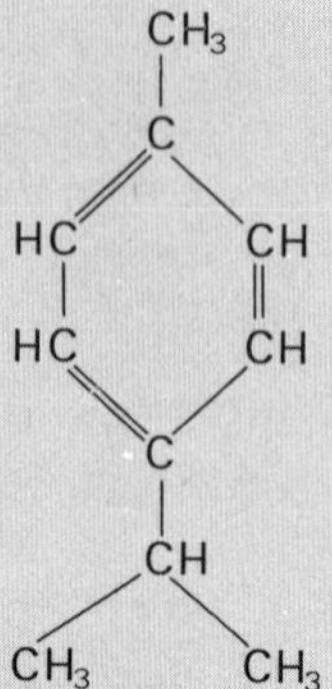

Cymene
(aromatic hydrocarbon)

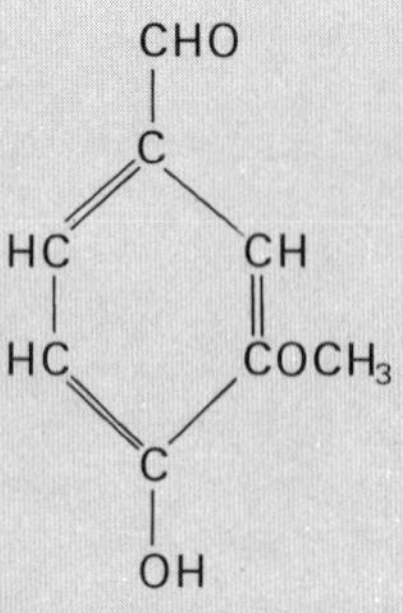

Vanillin
(aromatic aldehyde)

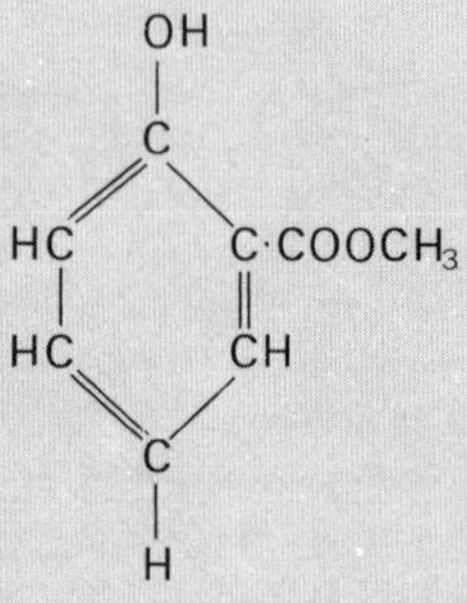

Methyl salicylate
(aromatic ester)

Table 5·4 Terpenes and related constitutents of volatile oils

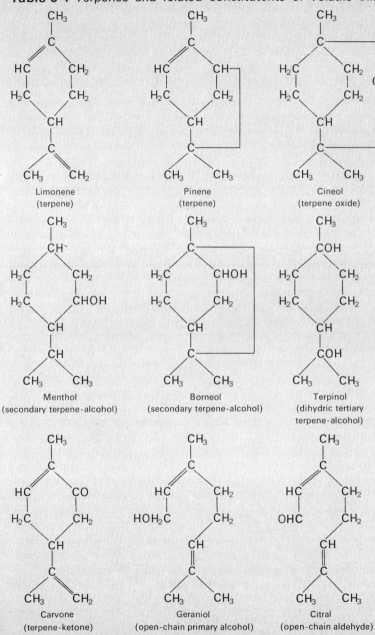

Limonene
(terpene)

Pinene
(terpene)

Cineol
(terpene oxide)

Menthol
(secondary terpene-alcohol)

Borneol
(secondary terpene-alcohol)

Terpinol
(dihydric tertiary
terpene-alcohol)

Carvone
(terpene-ketone)

Geraniol
(open-chain primary alcohol)

Citral
(open-chain aldehyde)

Spices

In one of the volumes of their classical compilation on food composition the Wintons wrote: 'Although flavour is an important
factor in making food more enjoyable, it is no more a mark of
nutritive value than colour in fabrics is a measure of durability'. In
fact, none of the large number of substances which, from the times
of the Spice Islands of history to this day, have been important
articles of trade, makes any significant contribution to food value.
Some, indeed, may be toxic.

Consider how remarkable is the commerce in these 'non-foods'
which are, as they have always been, esteemed for aesthetic rather
than nutritional reasons. This does not make them any the less
valued. In prisons, men will mortgage their future freedom and
sacrifice their friends for another 'non-food' that also occupies
good agricultural land, namely, tobacco. There is a lesson for food
scientists in both tobacco and spices (and, for that matter, in
onions). It is that food habits are a part of the total complex of
human behaviour.

Spices come from the most diverse botanical and geographical
origins. Lemon grass (*Cymbopogon citratus*), originally from the
East Indies, and citronella from Ceylon are leaves of the grass
family; calamus, the sweet flag from European swamps, is a
rhizome of the *Arum* family, while orris is the dried rhizome of the
iris family. The Zingiberaceae family provides ginger, thought to
have originated in tropical Asia, and turmeric, a native of India.
The stems and leaves of the laurel family contribute bay leaves as
well as sassifras, cinnamon, cassia and camphor. The mint family,
Labiatae, is the source of sweet basil, peppermint, Japanese mint,
water mint, spearmint, marjoram, thyme, rosemary, sage and clary.
Sweet basil comes originally from tropical Asia and Africa, peppermint is European, Japanese mint came from China and Korea as
well as Japan, water mint and spearmint are both European
although spearmint is grown extensively nowadays in Michigan and
New York, marjoram is Mediterranean as is rosemary and sage.

Clary (*Salvia sclarea* L.), is grown throughout southern Europe and the Orient.

And so the list goes on. The stem and leaves of Compositae provide tarragon from western Siberia. The iris family supplies saffron; capers come from the Capparidaceae. The myrtle family yields cloves – dried flower buds – from an evergreen tree native to the Moluccas; the pine family provides juniper berries. Vanilla comes from a vine with aereal roots; the plant is a native of Mexico. Pepper is the berry of a woody vine found growing native on the Malibar coast of India. Anise comes from a tree of the magnolia family originating in the Orient. Nutmeg and mace are produced by a tree of the Myristicaceae family from the Banda Islands in the Far East. Mustard is derived from widely distributed Cruciferae while fenugreek – popular with North African women, who believe it improves the figure, and used in America to simulate a maple flavour – belongs to the pea family

All these plants and more, with romantic names, gathered from the four corners of the earth, serve to remind the food scientist of the varied ramifications of his subject.

Part 2

Developments in the understanding of nutrition

6 The evolution of nutritional science

One of the earliest experimental studies in nutrition is that described in the first chapter of the Book of Daniel. There it is reported that Daniel persuaded Melzar, the officer appointed by King Nebuchadnezzar to look after the training of Daniel and his three companions, Shadrach, Meshach and Abed-nego, to carry out a trial to compare the nutritional value of a specially selected ration with the customary meals provided at court. The account runs as follows (vv 11–15): 'Then said Daniel to Melzar . . . prove thy servants, I beseech thee, ten days; and let them give us pulse to eat and water to drink. Then let our countenances be looked upon before thee, and the countenance of the children that eat of the portion of the king's meat . . . And at the end of ten days their countenances appeared fairer and fatter in flesh than all the children which did eat the portion of the king's meat.'

This is one example of an early writing in which the components of diet have been accepted as possessing an influence on health and fitness capable of being assessed by direct observation. There are others. One particularly interesting one can even be taken to imply that the effect of fish liver on the eye-disease, xerophthalmia – now known to be due to a deficiency of vitamin A – had been recognised in ancient times. The reference is in chapter 11 of the Book of Tobit in the Apocrypha. Tobias' father, Tobit, had become blind due to the development of a white film, which may well have been xerophthalmia, which had formed over his eyes. The angel, Raphael, who was advising Tobias during the course of his journey, had recommended him to preserve the liver of a fish he had caught. When they arrived at Tobit's house, he instructed Tobias: 'Take in thine hand the gall of the fish and . . . anoint his eyes with the gall . . . Tobit also went forth towards the door, and stumbled: but his son ran unto him . . . and strake the gall on his father's eyes, saying, Be of good hope, my father . . . And the whiteness pilled away from the corners of his eyes: and when he saw his son, he fell upon his neck.'

These examples of nutritional observation from early writings are unusual. For the most part, the ideas of the ancients about the

6·1 An alchemical diagram epitomising the ancient belief that everything, including different foods, was composed of mixtures of the four 'elements' : earth, air, fire and water. In consequence some foods 'cooled the blood' while others produced a 'fiery' temperament.

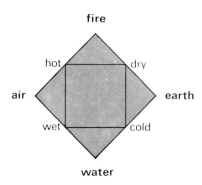

effect of different foods on health, just like those of primitive communities today, were almost completely illogical. This does not mean that they had no reason for their beliefs. Such reasons as they had, however, were derived from faith rather than from natural observation. From 1500 BC, in Egypt and India, and particularly at the time of Aristotle, it was believed that all matter was composed of the four elements, earth, air, fire and water, linked to the qualities dry, wet, hot and cold. Everything partook to varying degree of these qualities, including people's temperaments and the diseases they suffered. Consequently foods, too, were recommended on the basis of the degree to which they contributed to the allegedly desirable qualities of hotness, coldness, wetness or dryness.

Magic and religious beliefs exerted a strong influence and indeed continue to do so to this day. For example, certain people hold that red port wine 'makes blood' – because it is red. This dates back to the so-called 'doctrine of signatures'. This doctrine asserted that the colour or appearance of a food could indicate what function it exerted in the body after it had been eaten. Red food – beef for instance – contributed to blood formation, yellow foods would cure jaundice or, in some interpretations of the doctrine, would cause it. When potatoes were introduced into Europe, their pale, knobbly appearance and the strange way that they grew under the ground was taken to imply in some quarters that they would give anyone who ate them leprosy because this disease gives rise to a pale and roughened dermatitis.

An even more primitive idea was that by eating meat a man could acquire the characteristics of the creature from which it came. This was often the basis of cannibalism. A man would eat the heart of a gallant enemy in order that he might acquire his courage, or he would eat the flesh of a lion. On the other hand he would avoid chicken for fear of becoming timid. Some groups abstained from pork in fear of their eyes becoming small and close set. Others ate dog to acquire loyalty.

The science of nutrition as we know it today could begin only in the nineteenth century. This is because its foundation is built on the discoveries of the great Frenchman, Antoine Lavoisier. Only at the end of the eighteenth century and in his last productive years before his tragic death in the Revolution did he elucidate the nature of combustion, which, in principle, is the same process as respiratory oxidation by which man and the higher animals obtain the energy which keeps them alive. Certainly, there had been some acute observers before the 1790s but the basis to support a systematic scientific framework was wanting. As long ago as 1614, Sanctorius, in his book, *De medicina statica aphorismi*, published in Venice, described experiments in which he sat in a chair suspended from a large steelyard (a type of balance) and ate his dinner. When the yard dipped and he and the chair sank down, he stopped eating. Yet by the next meal, his weight was back to what it had been before. It was only in 1780 that Lavoisier measured the amount of 'insensible perspiration', by which weight was lost, recognised it as carbon dioxide and water and established that life was a chemical process – 'La vie est une fonction chimique' – and that the chemical compounds taking part in the process were derived from foods. From 1780 to 1920, the balance, the thermometer and the principles of chemistry were applied by a series of physiologists to establish in quantitative terms the energy relationships between food, work and the living body.

Lavoisier and Laplace made experiments on animal heat and respiration; the great German chemist, Liebig, received his early training in Paris before establishing his own laboratory where Voit, who died in 1908, carried out the painstaking researches which laid the foundations of the great nutrition school in Munich. Among his pupils were Rubner, Atwater and Lusk who established nutritional science in the United States, Cathcart whose work was done in Scotland, and many others.

The science of nutrition as we understand it today is made up of three main interwoven threads. The first, based firmly on Lavoisier's genius, is that life is a process of 'combustion' or, to put the same conception in a different way, that the energy by which a living creature is distinguished from a non-living one, is the product of the chemical combustion of fuel of some sort or another – that is food – with oxygen. This energy can be measured as heat, just as can the energy-value of coal, even though part of it is subsequently realised as movement or other work. The establishment of the energy relationships between different foods and the working of the body, together with the measurement of the efficiency with which the energy input can be converted into work output and, finally, the way in which an animal body may operate in equilibrium with its fuel supply, or may draw on banked fuel stocks in times of hardship, or, on the other hand, lay down fat and become obese – all these constitute the first main strand of nutritional science. The second has been the study of the way in which food provides not merely the energy to keep the biological 'machine' going, but also the basic structures of which it is built. The mobilisation of mineral elements to constitute the skeleton; iron and iodine for special biologically important molecules; and, perhaps most important of all, the nitrogen metabolism for the protein molecules constituting the muscular structure and the complex protoplasm of the body – these can all be taken to fall within this category.

And the third strand of scientific advance in the history of nutrition has been the striking advances achieved mainly within the present century, although with their roots coming from a few flashes of genius from earlier times, by which knowledge of vitamins and other so-called 'accessory food factors' has developed.

Energy

The first study by which the relationship between food and energy was established was that of Lavoisier and Laplace. They put a guinea-pig into a chamber surrounded by ice and measured the amount of ice melted in ten hours and the amount of carbon dioxide produced by the animal. Lavoisier, using a colleague, Sagiun, as an experimental animal, also measured the amount of oxygen absorbed as well as the amount of carbon dioxide produced and measured also by how much each was increased when measured amounts of physical work were done. These experiments, with no precedent behind them and carried out within a few months of the very discovery of oxygen by Joseph Priestley in England, were so excellently done and, even in the absence of sophisticated apparatus, the figures obtained were so accurate, that the principles Lavoisier established from them still stand today. For another hundred years after his death, that is throughout the nineteenth century, a series of distinguished physiologists elaborated the principles he had conceived. In France, Reynault and Reiset carried out numerous experiments on small animals in the 1840s, in Bavaria, Pettenkofer and Voit obtained the support of King Maximilian II for the construction of an elaborate chamber in which a man could live for several days and the oxygen he breathed in, the carbon dioxide and water breathed out and the heat he generated could all be measured – this was 1866. In Berlin, Switzerland and Sweden scientists established the framework upon which modern knowledge depends. Then, in 1892, Atwater, an American, who had been studying in Voit's laboratory in Munich, returned to the United States and, in collaboration with Rosa, an engineer, constructed a human 'calorimeter' with which it was possible to measure the heat produced by a man within an accuracy of 0·1 per cent. The machine incorporated the same type of gear for

6·2 The Atwater-Rosa-Benedict respiration calorimeter is a device by which the amount of heat produced by an animal can be precisely measured and at the same time the amount of oxygen used by the animal and the amount of carbon dioxide and water produced can also be measured.

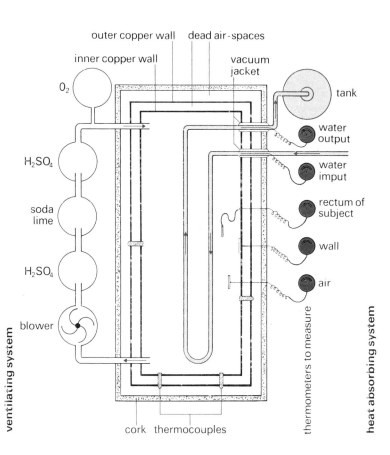

6·3 Below The Douglas bag is a device for collecting expired air. The proportions of oxygen and carbon dioxide in the air sample enable the metabolic activity to be calculated.
Right The Kofranyi-Michaelis respirometer being worn by a miner. This instrument is one of several that are useful in measuring the energy expenditure of industrial workers.

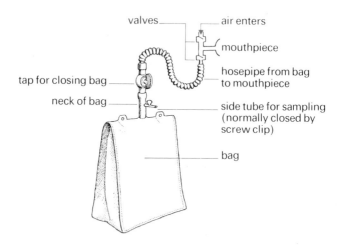

measuring gas exchange as that used by Pettenkofer and Voit.

This work was fundamental to nutritional science but when it had been done it became possible to shortcut its most severe technical difficulties. The fuel value of foods and their components had been established. It had been found that the energy released by carbohydrate (starch and sugar) and by fat was the same whether it was metabolised by a man's body or combusted in a calorimeter in the laboratory. Not all the chemical energy of protein was released in the body, however, because, it was discovered, the nitrogen was excreted in the form of the compound, urea, which still contained chemical energy which was not biologically utilisable by man (it does, however, yield its energy when fed to cows who make use of the micro-organisms in their rumen for the purpose). With this fundamental knowledge at hand, much useful information could be obtained without the need to make difficult measurements of heat. Instead, 'indirect' calorimetry could be done merely by measuring carbon dioxide output and oxygen input and relating them to the known calorific values of the food components – carbo-

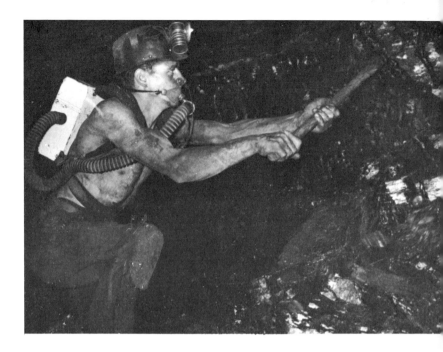

hydrate, fat or protein – from which they were derived.

As always, scientific advance inevitably being dependent on technique, knowledge advanced rapidly now that the manageably simple technique of 'indirect calorimetry' was available. The simplest type of apparatus was probably the 'Douglas bag', devised by the English scientist, Professor Douglas. This allows the gases breathed out while the individual being studied is taking part in various types of activity to be collected and the carbon dioxide and oxygen content of the total volume analysed later. By this means the expenditure of energy – measured in kilocalories – can be calculated for all sorts of work or for such activities as walking, walking upstairs or swimming. Since, if the person in question is not to lose weight, calories expended must be replaced by the food eaten, these measurements enable the requirements in terms of energy-value to be obtained.

More elaborate types of apparatus for making the same measurements are the Benedict-Roth 'spirometer' and the Max Planck respirometer, widely used in Germany. Another instrument which is

Table 6·1 Energy requirements for various activities (kilo-calories/hour)

Light work		Moderate work	
Sitting	19	Shoemaking	80–115
Writing	20	Sweeping	85–110
Standing relaxed	20	Dusting	110
Typing	16–40	Washing	125–215
Typing quickly	55	Charring	80–160
Sewing	30–90	Metal working	120–140
Dressing and undressing	33	Carpentering	150–180
Drawing	40–50	House painting	145–160
Lithography	40–50	Walking	130–240
Violin playing	40–50		
Tailoring	50–85		
Washing dishes	60		
Ironing	60		
Bookbinding	45–90		

Hard work		Very hard work	
Polishing	175	Stonemasonry	350
Joiner work	195	Sawing wood	420
Blacksmithing	275–350	Coal mining (average for shift)	320
Riveting	275	Running	800–1000
Marching	280–400	Climbing	400–900
Cycling	180–600	Walking very quickly	570
Rowing	120–600	Rowing very quickly	1240
Swimming	200–700	Running very quickly	1240
		Skiing	500–950
		Wrestling	1000
		Walking upstairs	1000

convenient for measuring the energy-expenditure of athletes or industrial workers is the Kofranyi-Michaelis respirometer. Table 6·1 shows the results of a number of these determinations.

Protein

The existence of proteins, or 'albuminous' substances as they were once called, as components of food in addition to fats and carbohydrates was recognised early in the history of nutrition. Pliny, for example, used the term *albumin* to describe the white of egg. And in more modern times, Macquer, in the edition of his dictionary published in 1777, used the word *albuminous* to include animal substances which coagulate when they are heated, for example, egg-white or blood serum, or indeed to describe animal matter in general. It was soon recognised that protein gave off ammonia when it was distilled – that is to say, that it contained nitrogen – and that vegetable foods also contained protein. Gluten from wheat flour, for example, had been recognised in the eighteenth century. And in 1843, Thomas Thomson reached the conclusion that 'animals are principally formed from the glutinous or albuminous principles of vegetables'.

Then, one by one, the components of which the protein molecules are constituted were discovered. Braconnot, a French chemist, in 1820 broke down the protein gelatin with sulphuric acid and from the syrup produced isolated the amino acid glycine. Then, from meat and from wool he prepared by a similar method a second, amino acid, leucine. In 1846, the German chemist Liebig prepared from the curds of milk – what would now be called casein – a third amino acid, tyrosine. The first sulphur-containing amino acid, cystine, was in fact prepared from urinary calculi – kidney stones – in 1810 but was only prepared from protein by Mörner in 1899. By this time the list was lengthening. So-called basic amino acids were isolated in 1886 (arginine), 1889 (lysine) and 1896 (histidine). Table 6·2 shows the sequence in which the more significant amino acids were discovered.

Table 6·2 Identification of the main nutritionally significant amino acids

Amino acid	Discoverer	Date	Amino acid	Discoverer	Date
Glycine	Braconnot	1820	Arginine	Hedin	1895
Leucine	Braconnot	1820	Histidine	Hedin, Kossel	1896
Tyrosine	Bopp	1849	Cystine	Mörner	1899
Serine	Cramer	1865	Valine	Fischer	1901
Glutamic acid	Ritthausen	1866	Proline	Fischer	1901
Aspartic acid	Ritthausen	1868	Tryptophan	Hopkins, Cole	1901
Phenylala-nine	Schulze, Barbiere	1881	Isoleucine	Ehrlich	1903
Alanine	Weyl	1888	Methionine	Mueller	1922
Lysine	Drechsel	1889	Threonine	Rose	1935

The discovery that proteins from different sources might differ in nutritional value was made by Lawes and Gilbert in England in 1854. They fed two pigs one on lentil meal and one on barley meal and observed that the one which depended on lentils for its protein lost more than twice as much of the nitrogen in the form of urea in its urine than the one obtaining its protein from barley. This implied that the one protein was more efficiently utilised than the other. But it was not until 1879 that it was appreciated that the nutritional value of a protein depended on the presence in its make-up of the appropriate combination of amino acids.

Some time previously, Magendie, the chairman of the Gelatin Commission set up by the Paris Academy, had observed that dogs could not thrive on a diet in which gelatin was the sole source of protein. Only after a great amount of work had been done by a number of investigators did the German workers, Hermann and Escher, hit on the idea of supplementing the gelatin with the amino acid tyrosine. They reported that when this was done, the loss of nitrogen from the body of the dogs which had been observed before was replaced by a gain. In fact, later studies showed that the main deficiency in the composition of gelatin was a lack of the sulphur-containing amino acid cystine.

This was the prelude to the conception of the 'biological value' of different proteins. Feeding trials with different types of animals (it is interesting to note that W.S. Savory, lecturer in anatomy at St Bartholomew's Hospital, London, appears to enjoy the distinction of being the first research worker to use rats in nutritional studies) were carried out and the 'biological value' of the particular protein under test was measured in terms of the degree to which it promoted growth in the experimental animal. The proteins of milk and eggs were found to be of high biological value while those of cereals and legumes were less good. It therefore came to be accepted by nutritionists that animal proteins were, in general, 'first-class' while those from vegetable sources were 'second-class'. This phase in the history of nutrition is perhaps best summed up by quoting from a paper by Crichton-Brown published in 1909 in which he wrote, 'The success of the races, their vitality and energy, might almost be measured by the degree to which animal flesh has entered into their diet.'

The next phase in the understanding of the nutritional significance of protein was directly dependent on the development of the technique of 'paper partition chromatography'. This method of analysis was invented by two young Englishmen, Martin and Synge, for which they were most appropriately awarded a Nobel Prize in 1952. Their technique made it possible, for the first time, to separate the constituent amino acids of a protein one from another. Previously, it had been a matter of prodigious difficulty to determine the amino acid make-up of different proteins. After this new and elegant procedure had been developed the time had arrived when nutritional requirements could be expressed, not in the loose qualitative terms of 'first-class' or 'second-class' protein but as the much more quantitative assessment of the need for a series of 'essential' amino acids of known chemical configuration. These were set out in table 2·2 on pp. 24 and 25.

Accessory food factors

In 1898, C.F. Langworthy, working for the US Department of Agriculture, summed up the scientific knowledge of nutrition thus: 'Foods have a dual purpose: building and repair. Energy for heat and work. Foods consist of the nutrients protein, fat and carbohydrates, and various mineral salts.' This level of knowledge was accepted as the whole of nutrition even up to the time of World War I in 1914. And as late as 1918, the British Ministry of Food in planning the national diet publicly condemned the use of fruit, tomatoes and vegetables as wasteful and unnecessary. Because their calorie values were low they were dismissed as being little better than coloured water in solid form. Similarly, because the importance of what even then was called vitamin A was not fully understood, the Danes exported most of their butter. This led to the appearance of xerophthalmia causing blindness among Danish children. A British garrison surrendered to the Turks at Kut in 1916, not because they did not have enough to eat but because they did not know that their supplies were deficient in B-vitamins and in vitamin C, enough of which could have been dropped to them from a single aeroplane even in those days to keep the defence going, if only there had been understanding then of what the American physiologist, McCollum, began to call 'accessory food factors'.

In 1753, James Lind, a Scottish naval surgeon, published an account of a carefully controlled experimental trial which he had done in 1747 during the course of a voyage on board a ship called the *Salisbury*. He showed that whereas seamen suffering from scurvy were in no way helped when treated with cyder, *elixir vitriol*, vinegar or half a pint of sea water a day – all of which were considered to be remedies – they were immediately and completely cured within six days when they were given two oranges and one lemon each day. The lesson of this clear-cut and dramatic demonstration was, however, not learned and, indeed, it was in later years forgotten. Among the first clear evidence for the existence in food

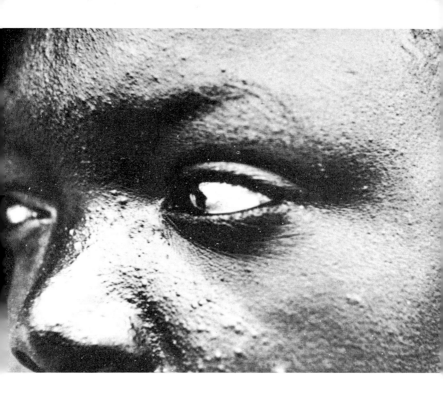

of constituents other than carbohydrate, protein, fat and minerals necessary in small amount for nutritional health was the investigation by the Dutch doctor, Eijkman, in 1896 in what were then the Dutch East Indies. He observed that chickens fed on a diet of polished rice developed the disease polyneuritis, which could be prevented or cured by the administration of rice polishings. Eijkman then had the genius to deduce that the human disease beri beri, which was widespread in the East, was also due to the consumption of polished rice and could be cured by an ingredient present in the discarded polishings.

But it was from the work of Pekelharing, carried out at the University of Utrecht in 1905, and that of Hopkins and his colleagues in the following year at Cambridge that the idea of accessory food factors, subsequently called 'vitamins', emerged. These researchers fed experimental mice and rats purified diets and observed that they failed to grow, but that growth was restored if

Table 6·3 Food and Nutrition Board, National Research Council recommended daily dietary allowances

	Age	Weight	Height	Kilo-calories	Protein
	Years	kg (lb)	cm (in)		g
Men	25	65 (143)	170 (67)	3,200	65
	45	65 (143)	170 (67)	2,900	65
	65	65 (143)	170 (67)	2,600	65
Women	25	55 (121)	157 (62)	2,300	55
	45	55 (121)	157 (62)	2,100	55
	65	55 (121)	157 (62)	1,800	55
Pregnant (3rd trimester)				Add 400	80
Lactating (850 ml daily)				Add 1,000	100
Infants	0–1/12				
	1/12–3/12	6 (13)	60 (24)	kg × 120	kg × 3·5
	4/12–9/12	9 (20)	70 (28)	kg × 110	kg × 3·5
	10/12–1	10 (22)	75 (30)	kg × 100	kg × 3·5
Children	1–3	12 (27)	87 (34)	1,200	40
	4–6	18 (40)	109 (43)	1,600	50
	7–9	27 (59)	129 (51)	2,000	60
Boys	10–12	35 (78)	144 (57)	2,500	70
	13–15	49 (108)	163 (64)	3,200	85
	16–20	63 (139)	175 (69)	3,800	100
Girls	10–12	36 (79)	144 (57)	2,300	70
	13–15	49 (108)	160 (63)	2,500	80
	16–20	54 (120)	162 (64)	2,400	75

Cal-cium	Iron	Vita-min A	Thia-mine	Ribo-flavin	Niacin	Ascor-bic acid	Vita-min D
g	mg	iu	mg	mg	mg	mg	iu
0·8	12	5,000	1·6	1·6	16	75	
0·8	12	5,000	1·5	1·6	15	75	
0·8	12	5,000	1·3	1·6	13	75	
0·8	12	5,000	1·2	1·4	12	70	
0·8	12	5,000	1·1	1·4	11	70	
0·8	12	5,000	1·0	1·4	10	70	
1·5	15	6,000	1·5	2·0	15	100	400
2·0	15	8,000	1·5	2·5	15	150	400
0·6	6	1,500	0·3	0·4	3	30	400
0·8	6	1,500	0·4	0·7	4	30	400
1·0	6	1,500	0·5	0·9	5	30	400
1·0	7	2,000	0·6	1·0	6	35	400
1·0	8	2,500	0·8	1·2	8	50	400
1·0	10	3,500	1·0	1·5	10	60	400
1·2	12	4,500	1·3	1·8	13	75	400
1·4	15	5,000	1·6	2·1	16	90	400
1·4	15	5,000	1·9	2·5	19	100	400
1·2	12	4,500	1·2	1·8	12	75	400
1·3	15	5,000	1·3	2·0	13	80	400
1·3	15	5,000	1·2	1·9	12	80	400

6 5 The lower curve shows the weight of Hopkins' rats fed on what had been thought to be a complete diet; they soon stopped growing and began to lose weight. Where the solid dots begin, a small amount of milk was fed to each rat and they at once began to grow. The upper graph shows the weights of another group which at first received doses of milk. Where the outline dots begin, the milk was stopped.

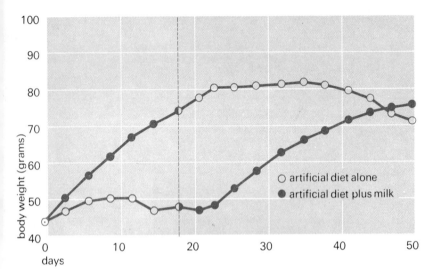

supplements of milk, far too small to contribute any significant amount of protein or calories, were added. From these beginnings an extensive series of substances have been identified, the chemical configuration of each elucidated and confirmed by synthesis, and in most instances its biochemical function determined. Those of most clearly recognised physiological significance are listed in table 6·4.

This brings us to the nutritional understanding of today. The composition of foods is known, at least so far as their content of nutrients is concerned. The calories they contribute, their content of carbohydrate, protein and fat, the mineral elements in them and the concentration of vitamins they contain have been determined. To be sure, there may be organic acids and pectins or compounds of obscure composition included in the omnibus term 'carbohydrate'; protein can be interpreted in terms of its amino acids but analysis of 'total protein' is often based on the analysis of nitrogen

Table 6·4 Vitamins of recognised physiological significance

1	Vitamin A	6	Pantothenic acid	11	Vitamin D
2	beta Carotene	7	Pyridoxin	12	Vitamin E
3	Thiamine	8	Biotin	13	Vitamin K
4	Riboflavin	9	Vitamin B_{12}	14	Folacin
5	Niacin	10	Ascorbic acid		

and may – and often does – include nitrogen-containing compounds other than protein; fats include a variety of fatty acids but also lipid compounds and so-called 'unsaponifiable fractions' including sterols. In short, when we assert that the composition of a particular foodstuff is known, we usually imply only that what we know about it is known. Prudent scientists will always leave open the possibility of there being something unknown still to be discovered.

In the same way, it is possible to set down the nutrient requirements for health of each category of individual, of men, women and children, of workers, expectant mothers and adolescents. In this sense, the modern understanding of nutritional science is epitomised in table 6·3.

7 Deficiency diseases

There are a number of people in the world who do not get enough to eat and who suffer accordingly. Such states can be divided into three groups. There are conditions due to a sheer lack of food; this is undernutrition. There are so-called deficiency diseases due to an imbalance of nutrients; these may be induced by the lack, for example, of one or more vitamins. And then there is ill-health due to amounts or proportions of nutrients unsuited to the circumstances of the particular consumer; obesity, ischaemic heart disease and conditions due to the consumption of too much of one or other nutrient can be included in this category.

Before considering examples of malnutrition from each of these groups, it is worth reflecting on the fact that, although a man dying of starvation or a patient suffering from beri-beri due to lack of thiamine, or goitre due to a shortage of iodine, can readily be recognised as suffering from a deficiency disease, there is a wide borderline area when, although it may be true that more or better food would improve a man's physical state, it is unreasonable to assert that he is ill or suffering for lack of it. In fact, it is not at all easy to define 'health'. Japanese men who live in California and eat a lavish American diet are, on average, taller and heavier than their relations who stay at home in Japan and eat traditional Japanese food. This does not imply that the native Japanese are malnourished. There have been great men who drew their strength from fasting and prayer. Nor does the definition of 'health' adopted by the World Health Organisation of the United Nations in 1946 resolve the situation for the nutritional scientist. It states that 'health is a state of complete physical, mental and social well-being and not merely the absence of disease and infirmity'.

Undernutrition

Many people have concerned themselves about the possibility of mass starvation. More important than this, however, is the gradual erosion of the vigour of a hard-pressed society. Among such populations, often in crowded urban areas dependent on the surrounding countryside for food, it is the poor and the helpless who suffer first. In a study of 278 families in Chile carried out in 1960, it was found that the average energy intake and protein consumption were 2,212 kilocalories and 68 g respectively. The poorest quarter of the people studied, however, were getting only 1,770 kilocalories and 50 g of protein. The same state of affairs was found in Brazil and in the Maharashtre State in India. Indeed in any place where the food supplies are inadequate the same state of affairs exists.

Children suffer first. The biological mechanism is such that the birth weight of babies born by undernourished mothers is frequently little less than those of well-fed women. But when children receive too little to eat, their growth is checked. It is not easy to determine, however, when undernutrition of this sort is permanently harmful. Every mother likes to see her children big for their age, that is to say, she likes them to grow quickly. There is little evidence, however, that, provided the period of food shortage is not unduly prolonged, the child may nevertheless develop into a well-grown, healthy adult. During and after the Second World War, a study of Belgian messenger boys showed that although their development was severely checked by malnutrition during the war years, they quickly caught up with their contemporaries when adequate food became available.

When too little food is available for adults, that is, when there is a shortage of calories, the first response of the body is a reduction in the *basal metabolic rate*. This implies that the vital processes 'tick over' at a slower rate. An individual, after losing a certain amount of weight and after his basal metabolism has fallen, may establish an equilibrium and live without undue distress in a permanent condition of 'undernutrition'. Many ascetics live all their lives and may achieve great things under these circumstances. Should a food shortage become severe, however, and famine supervene, the tissues of the body waste away, the skin becomes loose, the skeletal muscles atrophy as do the viscera and the heart. Only the tissues of the brain remain unaffected. Under these conditions a man may lose twenty-five per cent of his body weight,

7·1 **Right** The typical inelastic conditions of the legs of a sufferer from hunger oedema. When the leg is pressed with the finger, a 'dent' remains afterwards.
7·2 **Far right** A child suffering from kwashiorkor – one of the most common effects of protein deficiency. The more obvious symptoms of the complaint are wasting, oedema and skin lesions.

including the loss of 27 per cent of his body protein, 72 per cent of his fat and 9 per cent of the minerals from his bones as well. But in spite of these losses of body structure, the volume of circulating liquid, the so-called 'extracellular water' remains substantially unchanged. Sometimes, indeed, the water puffs up the features of a starving man who is lying down so that an unreceptive onlooker might not realise his predicament. When he stands up, however, this water collects in his legs, giving them the thick, puffy, inelastic condition characteristic of *hunger oedema*.

One of the most serious effects of starvation, the most serious of all deficiency diseases, is the thinning of the whole digestive tract. It can happen that the loss of elasticity and permeability may become so severe that, even if food supplies are restored, the unfortunate victim is unable to absorb nourishment so that his condition continues to deteriorate until he dies.

To summarise, it can be said that undernutrition may range from a temporary check in the growth rate of children, the harmfulness of which is hard to assess (there is no clear evidence that children that grow more *quickly* than their fellows become healthier adults), or the so-called 'low living' which is often associated with 'high thinking' in adults, through a gradual increase in adversity all the way to extreme privation and famine.

Protein deficiency

The most striking deficiency disease due to a combined lack of protein and calories in children, which has unfortunately been found in Africa, Central and South America and in certain other parts of the world, is *kwashiorkor*. This is primarily caused by a deficiency of amino acids and occurs in children shortly after weaning. It often occurs if the child first becomes the victim of an acute infection. The disease shows itself by muscular wasting, oedema, and failure to grow. Sometimes there is damage to the liver as well.

Where there is no recognisable 'disease', shortage of protein

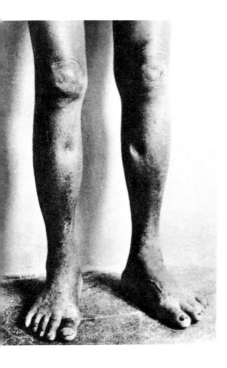
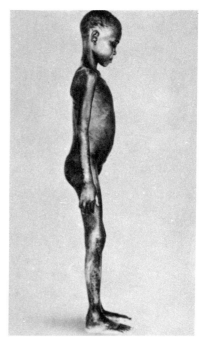

among children will restrict their growth. In adolescents or adults it may be a contributory cause of nutritional anaemia.

In 1963, it was estimated in the Third World Food Survey of the Food and Agriculture Organisation of the United Nations that one in five of all the populations of the less developed areas of the world was undernourished. By the very way it is stated, this figure can be seen to represent only a broad estimate, inevitably hardly more than an informed opinion. Similar estimates suggest that from 1 to 10 per cent of the children up to five or six years of age in the same parts of the world are affected by kwashiorkor or its variant, marasmus, a combined protein-calorie deficiency disease.

Scurvy – the disease of vitamin C deficiency

Although scurvy is a disease of considerable antiquity it is comparatively rare, in spite of the substantial number of underfed and malnourished people there are in the world. Scurvy, in fact, only

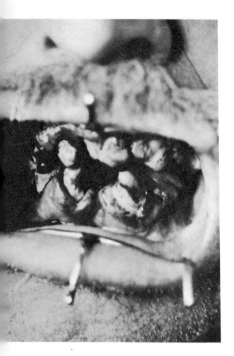
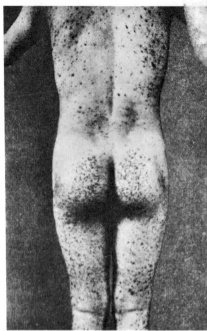

arises under rather peculiar conditions of deprivation. It was once common in the springtime after the long months of winter in the countries of northern latitudes before potatoes were introduced from South America. This can be readily understood now that scurvy is known to be due to a prolonged lack of fresh fruit and vegetables. But its ravages were most severe during the age of long sea voyages in sailing ships when the diet of the sailors was made up of items most easily preserved on board ship, namely, biscuits and salt pork. Arctic explorers were also subject to scurvy for the same reason.

It is only because of an unlucky biochemical fault in his genetical make-up that man is susceptible to the disease at all. The substance, ascorbic acid (vitamin C), is essential to the functioning of the cellular units of the tissues. Its role is to enable the amino acid proline to be converted into hydroxy-proline which is built up into the substance collagen, which acts as the cement by which cells are held together. This is why one of the symptoms of scurvy is a

7·3 Left A typical case of war-time scurvy in France 115
caused by vitamin C deficiency. The red spots are effused blood.
Far left Typical inflammation of the gums as a result of scurvy. This
complaint still exists today, even in well-developed countries,
due to eating no fruit and vegetables.

failure of wounds to heal and the tendency for old scars of long-healed injuries to burst open. Almost all the animals on earth synthesise ascorbic acid in their tissues. For this reason, the carnivores, the hoofed ungulates, dogs, cats, rats, mice – the list is almost all-embracing – are *not* subject to scurvy. This list covers almost all animals, but not quite. A few species are subject to an 'inborn error of metabolism'. They cannot synthesise vitamin C and so, if they fail to obtain enough ready-made from their food, they suffer from scurvy. These defective animals are the guinea pig, the red-vented bul-bul bird, the fruit-eating bat, the higher apes – and man.

Although scurvy, once common under the special circumstances of shipboard or siege or in isolated communities at the end of a long winter, is comparatively rare under modern conditions, it does nevertheless occur. It may occur among infants fed on artificial diets, perhaps made up of boiled milk in which all traces of vitamin C have been lost, and not given orange juice or another source of the vitamin. The children fail to thrive, many cry continuously because of haemorrhages in their joints and swollen and sore gums. Such scurvy was reported in recent years in Toronto in Canada, in several towns in India and in Glasgow in Scotland. Adult scurvy may also be seen, for example, so-called 'bachelor scurvy' may occur in older men living alone who neglect to provide cooked meals for themselves containing vegetables.

Beri-beri – the disease of thiamine deficiency

Beri-beri, which has been a scourge of the East from which thousands of people have died, is almost entirely a disease of the age of industrialisation. It appeared only after modern milling technology had been introduced from the West and marched across Asia producing polished rice for poor people at a cheaper price than that for which home-pounded rice could be provided. And in many African countries, refined white flour became popular and brought with its cheapness and palatability the same price in the disease of beri-beri.

7·4 Bizarre brothers: the guinea pig, the fruit-eating bat, the red-vented bul-bul bird, the anthropoid ape and man — the only five species of animal that need vitamin C in their food.

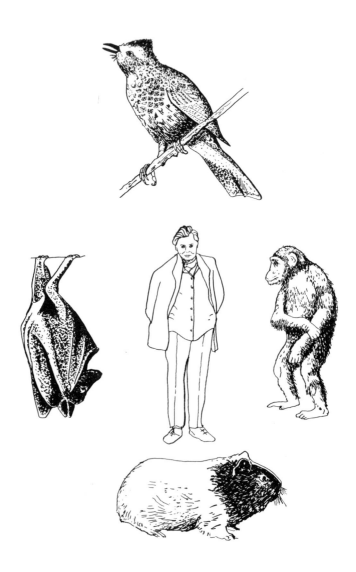

Beri-beri first occurred as an epidemic disease in the Japanese navy of the nineteenth century. The naval surgeon, Takaki, reported in 1879 nearly two thousand cases among five thousand men, the main part of whose rations was polished rice. It has since been found in China, Malaya, Indonesia, Singapore, parts of India, and in the Philippines. The disease takes three forms: 'wet beri-beri' is accompanied by oedema (dropsy), palpitations, breathlessness and muscular pain. Death, if it comes, is due to acute circulatory failure accompanied by extreme breathlessness. 'Dry beri-beri' is apparent as wasting, emaciation and weakness. Death may sometimes follow the sudden onset of oedema or an attack of dysentery. The third variant of beri-beri affects infants; the victim may suddenly die of heart-failure. In some cases a premonitory sign is when the infant's cry becomes thin and faint and it unsuccessfully attempts to cry.

Beri-beri, whatever form it takes, is always due to lack of the vitamin thiamine in the diet. Yet there is no unanimity about the best means of preventing it. The vitamin can quite readily be synthesised in a chemical factory and sold at a low price. Some authorities advocate the addition of such synthetic material to polished rice and white flour. Other authorities consider it better to modify the technological process by which vitamin-deficient polished rice and white flour are manufactured so that, for example, 'parboiled' rice and flour of increased 'extraction rate' containing increased concentrations of thiamine will become available.

The appearance of ill-health due to a deficiency of thiamine, although basically due to a shortage of the vitamin, is affected by several other factors. First of all, the need for thiamine is greatest when a diet rich in sugar and starch is eaten. Consequently, deficiency symptoms are most likely when polished rice is the main article of diet. In Western populations, white flour and sugar are equally dangerous. Perhaps vitamin-deficiency symptoms among adults in the West are commonest among alcoholics. This is partly because the energy value from alcohol is not supported by any intake of thiamine. A second cause of alcoholic neuritis due to thiamine deficiency is the poor diet of many heavy spirit drinkers.

But there are some curious additional causes of thiamine deficiency. There is in certain uncooked fish an enzyme, thiaminase, capable of destroying thiamine. It has been found that people who eat uncooked clams may reduce the effective amount of thiamine which they would otherwise obtain from the rest of their diet by 50 per cent. This enzyme has also been identified in ferns and in certain bacteria, although this is of little significance in human nutrition.

Pellagra – the disease mainly due to niacin deficiency

The disease, pellagra, is a gift to mankind, if gift it can be called, by which the Red Indians of the New World, exterminated by the colonists from the Old World, have in a small measure repaid the compliment. Of all the plants brought from the Americas, not excluding tobacco, maize was most eagerly adopted and rapidly spread across Europe and Asia. And pellagra has occurred all over the world wherever maize has become a staple cereal. It has been a scourge among poor people in Spain, Italy and France, in Yugoslavia, Rumania, Bulgaria and the Ukraine. Epidemics have occurred in Egypt and other parts of North Africa. And in the Southern States of North America it was, until recent years, a serious public health problem.

It is now clear that pellagra is due to a shortage of the vitamin niacin in the diet. But this deficiency is complicated by the fact that the amino acid tryptophan possesses the same sort of vitamin activity. The fact that the concentration of niacin and of tryptophan in foods varies and that their availability to the body may also vary from one food to another makes it difficult to evaluate the pellagra-preventative – that is, the vitamin-equivalent – effect of different foods. It is generally accepted nowadays, however, that approximately 60 mg of tryptophan is equivalent to 1 mg of niacin in its vitamin effect. The reason why a diet predominantly made up of maize is conducive to pellagra is because maize is relatively deficient in both niacin and tryptophan.

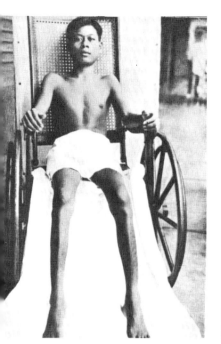

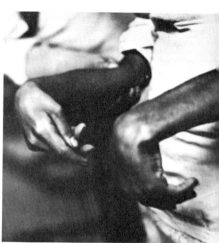

7·5 Two symptoms of beri-beri: wrist drop and wasting of the legs.

People whose diet is critically lacking in niacin or in tryptophan or both and who develop pellagra are almost always poor. It is their poverty that impels them to live on the limited food supply that is their downfall. In the southern United States, the traditional pellagra-producing diet was maize – corn, as it is called in America – molasses and a little salt pork. Pellagra sufferers are generally underweight. But the commonest sign of the disease is an affection of the skin resembling severe sunburn. This is usually symmetrically disposed on those parts exposed to the sun – on the face, the backs of the hands, the wrists and forearms. The mouth becomes sore and the tongue acquires an appearance like raw beef and becomes red, swollen and painful. As well as this, the whole of the gastro-intestinal tract may become inflamed, causing diarrhoea. As the disease proceeds, nervous symptoms appear. The patients become anxious, depressed and irritable. Later they may be delirious, lose their sense of touch and are unable to walk due to nervous lesions causing foot-drop. It can thus be seen that there is justification for

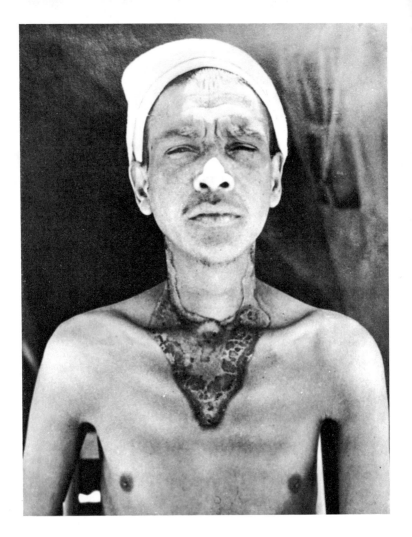

the common summary used to describe the effects of pellagra: dermatitis, diarrhoea and dementia. All this may be dramatically cured – sometimes within 24 hours – by the administration of 100 mg of niacin at, say, 4-hourly intervals.

Whenever a new factor is introduced into the dietary habits of a community, the consequences are complex. Maize is a valuable

7·6 A case of pellagra, due to deficiency
of niacin or to a combined deficiency of niacin
and the amino acid tryptophan.
A common symptom shown here –
Casal's necklace – resembles severe sunburn.

121

foodstuff. It was the staple cereal of the Red Indians of North America whose methods of culturing it in the fields and preparing the grain for use were adopted by the European and Asian nations who accepted it. Yet the consequences for them in the urban communities in which they lived were very different from the pastoral tribes of the American Indians whose food it had been; pellagra occurred. The adoption of the potato, another American introduction, as the main foodstuff for another impoverished European population, the Irish, was also followed in due time by disastrous consequences when, after a series of wet years, this crop showed its deficiency, on this occasion a susceptibility to infection. In our own time, we too are introducing a new factor into our food supply, so-called food technology. We would be prudent if we remembered the lessons of beri-beri and pellagra and reflected carefully on all the implications which this innovation may bring in its turn.

Rickets – the disease due to vitamin D deficiency

Rickets is a deficiency disease occurring in infancy and early childhood due primarily to a shortage of vitamin D in the diet. The chemical composition of the different variants of vitamin D are known; the vitamin can, indeed, be synthesised and, in fact, large amounts are made in this way by the pharmaceutical industry. The biochemical function of vitamin D has also been largely elucidated: it serves to enable calcium, the main constituent of bones and teeth, to be absorbed from the gut and thus made available to the body. It has also been discovered that vitamin D is required by most vertebrate species and that it can be made available to an animal – or to the human infant – either as the preformed vitamin in the diet or by the action of the ultra-violet light of the sun. The ultra-violet rays convert the natural sterols of the skin into the active form of the vitamin. Studies have been made of these and a variety of other attributes of vitamin D. For example, experiments with chickens have shown that these creatures require approximately the same amount of vitamin D in proportion to their body weight as babies do, and yet chickens very rarely develop rickets under normal circumstances. The explanation for this anomaly which is now accepted is that the birds obtain enough vitamin D for their needs from the oils they acquire from their own preen gland when preening themselves.

Yet in spite of all this detailed biochemical information, rickets in real life is only partly a biochemical phenomenon. This is a general lesson which food scientists have to learn about vitamin D, as about many other aspects of their subject. Rickets is a disease of poverty. It occurs among the children of the poor whose parents cannot afford to buy milk for them and whose houses are dark and, perhaps, huddled together in dark narrow streets in smoky sunless parts of crowded cities.

Rickets is today a comparatively rare disease. In the latter part of the last century, up to 75 per cent of the children of the poorer classes living in industrial cities had rickets. Glasgow in Scotland, Vienna in Austria, and Lahore in India were all notorious as places where the disease was rife.

The infant with rickets is not necessarily underfed; it may indeed receive too much cereal and sugar to eat. It is not unknown for the solid fat child that sits so still and is apparently contented to be selected as the winner of a baby show even though it is suffering from rickets. Yet such a baby will be fretful, with flabby toneless muscles and a distended abdomen. But the most profound effect of the disease is on the formation of the bones. When the rachitic child begins to walk, the shafts of its leg bones may become deformed and it develops knock-knees or bow-legs. Its spine may become deformed as well and so may its pelvis. In girls, this deformity may later on lead to serious difficulties in childbirth.

The virtual disappearance of rickets in those countries in which adequate steps have been taken to improve the conditions of the poor and use the knowledge nutritional science provides has been due to a variety of causes. Among these are improved housing and the provision of proper diet, particularly milk. Lastly, there has

7·7 Severe rickets due to vitamin D deficiency in undernourished 6-year olds. The centre child is nearly normal.

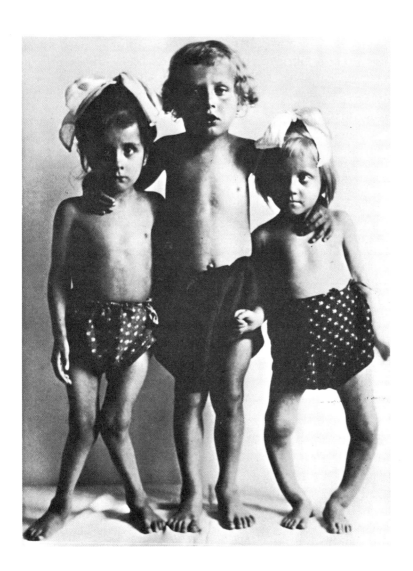

7·8 Right An advanced stage of thyroid enlargement due to iodine deficiency. This case comes from the Belgian Congo, where goitre is endemic.
7·9 Far right Riboflavin deficiency often results in pigmentary changes in the skin, particularly at the corners of the mouth, as shown here.

been the supply of vitamin D and, as in Great Britain, the fortification of bread with calcium. But although rickets is primarily due to the lack of vitamin D, the supplementation of articles of diet with the vitamin has led to certain consequences other than those intended and shows once again that human nutrition needs knowledge comprising more than just biochemistry.

Because vitamin D is cheap to manufacture, it has been added to different kinds of food. Among these are dried milk mixtures intended for feeding babies, margarine, cocoa, chocolate mixes and cereal preparations. The daily needs of an infant for vitamin D are about 400 international units, and yet it has been calculated that the actual amount consumed in a technologically orientated country such as the United States or Canada may exceed 4,000 iu. This may lead to overdosage. Indeed, in the 1950s in Great Britain, where the provision of vitaminised dried milk for infants together with a number of other measures had already done away with rickets, another disease, 'ideopathic hypercalcaemia' began to appear. This, in its turn disappeared only after the level at which the dried milk powder was fortified with vitamin D had been reduced.

There are a number of other nutritional deficiency diseases in addition to those which I have so far described. Anaemia may be caused by a lack of available iron in the diet. Lack of either of the vitamins vitamin B_{12} or folic acid may also lead to anaemia. Both these substances are concerned with the formation of blood, which takes place in the bone marrow. Anaemia also occurs in patients suffering from scurvy. It follows that anaemia in underfed people may be the result of insufficient vitamin C (ascorbic acid) even if the lack has been insufficiently severe to produce recognisable scurvy. A deficiency of one further vitamin, vitamin B_6 (pyridoxin) may also, though rarely, be the cause of anaemia.

But in real life and under normal circumstances, malnutrition is not necessarily recognisable as a specific deficiency disease. First, a community is never a homogeneous collection of uniform people. Always, some members of a society of people are richer and more fortunate than others. Even in times of severe hardship, some

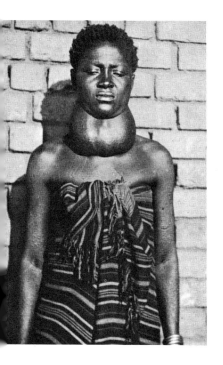
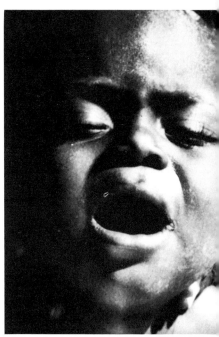

people will have enough to eat, just as it is equally true that in rich and prosperous communities – in the United States or Sweden – there will be those who are unfortunate, poor and malnourished. Then again, in a population of mixed ages and sexes there are always vulnerable groups, the very young and the very old, widows with large families, and those under the stress of ill-health or injury.

Furthermore, just as the community represents a spectrum of social classes and physiological status, so also is an inadequate diet rarely deficient in one single nutrient. It follows that malnutrition is commonly a partial lack of several nutrients, and the deviation from health that it causes is a mixed deficiency rather than a clear-cut text-book deficiency disease. There are few communities to be found whose diets, if analysed and converted into terms of nutrients, would provide for all their members the optimum amounts shown in table 6·3. When the state of health of such people, who are, in arithmetical terms, nutritionally deficient, is carefully examined, gradually, as their degree of deficiency becomes more severe, a

7·10 Obesity is malnutrition just as is undernutrition. This 31 stone man took part in a weight competition, and won the first prize of 31 stone of sugar! Statistically, the life-span of such fat men is greatly shortened.

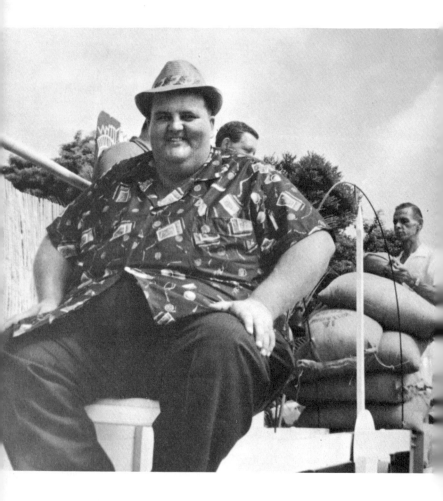

number of signs and symptoms, at first vague but later more definite, will be observed.

Lack of protein of the appropriate amino-acid make-up will stunt children's growth; too little to eat – that is, lack of calories – will lead to underweight and loss of vigour. Shortage of iron, B-vitamins and vitamin C will, as I have just described, lead to anaemia. Insufficient riboflavin may produce soreness at the corners of the mouth and a peculiar 'bloodshot' state of the eyes. Insufficient vitamin A can cause, first, night-blindness (hemeralopia) and, if prolonged, xerophthalmia. Affections of the skin, of the tongue, changes of the hair and nails, may be indicative of malnutrition. All these early indications of nutritional deficiency can be identified by a skilled observer; to attribute them with certainty to dietary deficiency, biochemical analysis of blood must also be carried out.

Deficiency diseases can be disastrous. People have died painful and distressing deaths from scurvy, pellagra and beri-beri. Children have grown up stunted and deformed by rickets or been blinded by xerophthalmia from lack of vitamin A. To eat a diet containing significantly less of the various nutrients listed in table 6·3 than the amounts shown may induce the less well defined symptoms I have just described. But to miss one's dinner, although it is to suffer dietary deficiency, causes no permanent harm and men have done great deeds under conditions of privation. And should the pendulum swing too far and a man eat too much, again he lays himself open to malnutrition. In many Western countries, obesity is widespread and more lives are shortened by obesity than by any other nutritional disorder. Diabetes and, particularly, coronary heart disease are also clearly attributable to dietary surplus.

The proper application of nutritional science calls for a balanced judgment equally as for a balanced diet.

8 Starvation

The particular interest in the topics of food science and nutrition today is that we know that there are people in the world who do not have enough to eat. We know also that the number of people in the world is increasing and, although this is less easy to assess in view of the great advances in agricultural science which are taking place as well, there is a chance that supplies of food are not keeping pace with the increase in population. It is common to meet people who are concerned that a proportion of the world's inhabitants is starving, and from time to time estimates are put forward of how many starving people there may be. I propose, therefore, in this chapter to discuss the nature of starvation.

Famine and starvation are not new. History is full of references to famines, and literature from the earliest times contains the most graphic accounts of them. Although it is the purpose of this book to describe food and its function or the lack of it in nutritional terms, it must always be remembered that the science of human nutrition is only one part of the total human situation. Starvation and famine rarely exist as isolated phenomena. Famine is almost always interlinked with disease. And the lack of food is commonly accompanied by raised prices. In July 1197, during a time of famine, the records kept by Reiner of Lüttich show that the price of a modius of rye was 40 solidi. Three years later, when plenty had returned, the price was 3·5 solidi. In 1891, during the great Russian famine, the peasants died of starvation, and yet rye bread could be bought freely in Novo Terenka for three farthings a pound; only the landless peasants had no money. In the Irish famine during the nineteenth century, food could be bought and the hotels were open, although the poor people were dying in thousands in the streets and in their cottages.

On 17 September 1944, the Dutch railwaymen declared a strike as part of their struggle against the forces occupying their country. In retaliation, the German military authorities cut off all supplies of food to Western Holland. From November 1944 to the following May there was famine during which people died of starvation. The Dutch are a civilised, highly educated nation and, being fully aware of the nutritional significance of the disaster with which they were faced, were able, while suffering, as all mankind must suffer when famine strikes, to observe and record the facts of their situation. The Dutch famine of 1944–5 is therefore particularly instructive to those who wish to understand the nature of starvation.

Before the Second World War (as afterwards), the people of the Netherlands enjoyed a satisfactory level of nutrition due in part to their prosperous agriculture and high level of technological industry and in part as well to their understanding of nutritional science, to which, indeed, Dutch research workers have made significant contributions. Importation of food ceased immediately after the German occupation in May 1940. Furthermore, approximately 60 per cent of the agricultural production of Holland was requisitioned by the occupying forces. Nevertheless, by dint of ploughing up pasture land to grow potatoes and slaughtering large numbers of pigs and poultry, the Dutch authorities were able to maintain food distribution at a level sufficient to contribute an average of between 1,600 and 1,800 kilocalories a day from 1941 until the summer of 1944. This represented hardship but not starvation. A well-judged rationing scheme was imposed so that heavy workers got more and mothers and children received their special needs. When food supplies were cut off in the winter of 1944–5 the total amount of food available for distribution quickly fell to about 600 kilocalories a day. By January 1945 it became no longer possible to give workers larger rations than ordinary people although efforts were still made to protect as far as possible infants, young children and expectant and nursing women.

The extent to which people could supplement their rations inevitably varied a good deal. Those living in the towns were worse off than the country people, and the poor and the old were worst off of all. The cold weather added to the people's hardships and hampered the distribution of what food there was. Sugar-beets from the fields were rationed and in some towns even tulip bulbs were included as part of the food issue. People went as best they could with bicycles and perambulators from the towns to the countryside in search of food. A few potatoes or sugar-beets were treasure. Anything that could be eaten was sought after. Before long, the cold of the winter and the failing strength of the people made these desperate efforts unavailing. Many died from exhaustion by the roadside. The old, particularly, suffered badly.

The Dutch medical authorities studied the composition of the diet available to the population during the winter of famine. In the main, the food, such as it was, contained significant proportions of the various vitamins. The deficiency was lack of calories, that is to say, there was not enough to eat and so the people starved. Until September 1944, in spite of wartime rationing, the general health of the population was good, although some loss of weight had been noticed and there were signs that the incidence of tuberculosis was beginning to rise. But as soon as food supplies were cut off people began to lose weight, they quickly tired whenever they had to exert themselves and complained of feeling cold. Starvation is known to affect people's minds and these people in Holland became mentally listless, apathetic and constantly obsessed with thoughts of food.

By January 1945, in the fourth month of the famine, the first cases of hunger oedema appeared and were admitted to hospital. Soon the numbers multiplied. Little could be done, however, because even in the hospitals there was no food to give. Indeed, all that the doctors and nurses had to eat themselves was one slice of bread for breakfast, two potatoes and a little vegetable with watery sauce for their midday meal, and one or sometimes two slices of bread, a plate of sugar-beet soup and a cup of coffee-substitute for supper. By February, there were so many starvation patients that the hospitals could no longer take them. The best that could be done was to give the worst sufferers – defined as those who had lost 25 per cent of their body-weight or more – supplementary rations of 400 g of bread and 500 g of beans a day with a little milk, if there was any, and discharge them as soon as they could walk.

As conditions deteriorated, the criterion by which patients received supplementary food became more stringent. Instead of being entitled to it when they had lost 25 per cent of their normal weight, the figure was raised to 33 per cent. Now people dropped from exhaustion in the streets and many died there. Others, who had made their way to treatment centres for help, were too weak to get home and took shelter in barns or wherever they could. Others again, who lacked the strength to go searching for food or help, stayed in bed and there they died.

The famine was accompanied by all its historical consequences – and this in civilised Holland in the twentieth century. Vermin became common; there was no soap – fat could not be spared to make it. Many people had skin infections and abscesses. In the main, the nutritional state of infants was well maintained. Some starved infants did, however, die, often when their parents had sold the coupons which were issued to provide them with special food: and this, too, is a result of famine and its effect on human behaviour. Then, outbreaks of dysentery occurred; in some rural districts waterborne typhoid broke out and there were no disinfectants to check it, just as there was no soap. Because of the shortage of fuel, several families would move into one house to keep warm. Gangs broke into the empty houses and carried off furniture and doors for fuel. The waiting room at Rotterdam station was thus looted one night. And people were injured and some killed when the walls or roofs of houses they were ransacking fell in on them.

In the four cities of Amsterdam, Rotterdam, The Hague and Utrecht, whereas in the first six months of 1939 the number of people in the populations who died were 3,655, 2,616, 2,419, and 776, in the six famine months of 1945 the numbers dying were 9,735, 7,827, 6,458 and 2,065, an increase of nearly 18,000 in a population of just over two million. Table 8·1 shows what the hospitals who tried to deal with starvation found about the loss of weight suffered by the people who came to them. It must be remembered that only when 25 per cent (later raised to 33 per cent) of weight had been lost was any help given, so severe was the food shortage. When weight loss reached about 40 per cent, it was too late to help and the people died.

The most obvious signs of starvation were extreme emaciation,

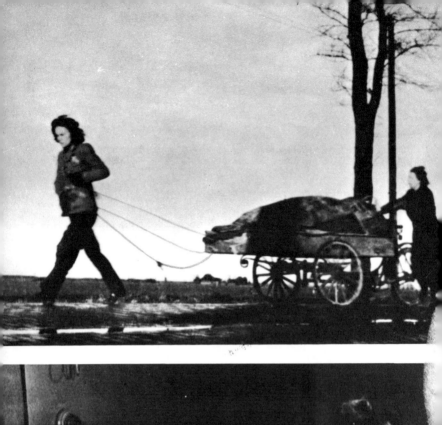
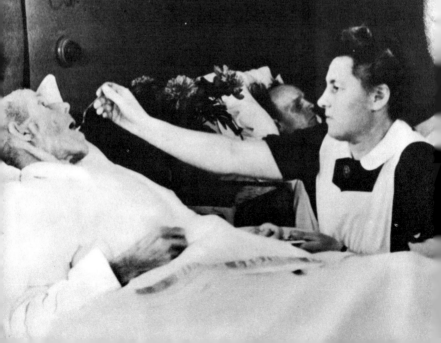

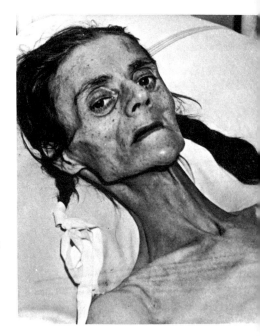

8·1 Top left By January 1945 the Dutch famine was in its fourth month. Those who had not the strength to pack their bags and go searching for food went home to bed and died.
Bottom left A case of starvation being looked after in a Dutch hospital in 1945. Soon the hospitals became too full to take any more.
Right A starving Dutch woman in bed, too weak to call for help.

hollow jaws, sunken eyes, wasted limbs and prominent ribs. The skin of the victims was sallow, often showing a characteristic dun-brown colour, either all over or on just the exposed areas. It was often dry and scaly. People quite often had chilblains and older victims frequently had skin haemorrhages.

In the Dutch famine, as in many others reported in the literature, a sign that made the greatest impression on the doctors was hunger-oedema. This was most often seen in the region of the ankles or in the face. Sometimes it was severe, extending right up the legs to the abdomen. It might be thought, mistakenly, that these sufferers had not lost weight, so great was the quantity of liquid with which they were encumbered. Both head lice and body lice as well as scabies were common. Starving people complain of feeling cold and, in fact, they often are cold. Temperatures below 33°C were found and were sometimes even as low as 27°C. The mouth and throat of these severely undernourished people tended to be pale. Their tongues were sometimes sore; when patients had diarrhoea, as a number had, their tongues were dry and furred.

The famine was brought about when food was cut off from West Holland in September 1944. It was terminated when food supplies were brought in by the relieving armies in May 1945. As the friendly troops marched in, all the people who were able came out into the streets to rejoice. It is an important fact that some of those who saw the cheering crowds were surprised and disbelieved the reports of starvation they had heard. The figure for the number of dead and the evidence of figure 8·1 underline how fallible such conclusions may be. But the joyful gaiety was itself a fact about famine that in any human situation there is always a gradation of physiological status. Furthermore, nutrition must always be interpreted within the context of the complex by which human behaviour is determined. The ecstatic people in the streets of liberated western Holland looked thin but flushed with emotion and excitement. 'We had expected,' wrote the reporter of the London *Times*, 'to find the most horrible conditions . . . but we did not need the special teams which stood by ready for action . . . There were some cases of advanced malnutrition, but no cases of actual starvation'. The 18,000 dead from hunger in the four big towns and the rows of pitiful patients, some of the many hundreds under treatment for starvation and hunger oedema in the wards of the hospitals, were not there cheering in the streets.

The famine accompanied by starvation which overtook the Dutch in 1944–5 was an example of a nutritional disaster, which had a clear cause, a definite beginning and a firmly marked end. The famine which occurred in Ireland almost exactly one hundred years earlier had very much more complex beginnings and illustrates, even if in rather a different way, the subtle interaction of influences which combine to produce nutritional results. It is a very much mistaken over-simplification to assert, without qualification, that people starve because they do not have enough to eat.

In the years 1845, 1846 and 1847 there was famine in Ireland and, so far as estimates are available, about one and a half million people starved to death or died of typhus or relapsing fever, disseminated by lice. Yet the causes of the famine and the starvation

Table 8·1 Weight lost by starvation patients

	Age	1940 weight	Weight recorded	Weight loss
		kilos	kilos	%
Patients	52	65	53	18
who recovered	47	64	52	19
	70	70	54	23
	66	80	61	24
	52	74	54	27
	71	73	54	27
	39	55	40	27
	73	72	52	29
	64	70	47	32
	61	78	49	36
	66	95	59	38
	69	68	42	38
	48	79	50	38
	85	85	49	42
	77	75	43	42
Patients	81	75	46	37
who died	71	72	40	44
	68	69	38	45
	68	76	40	47
	85	80	37	54
	40	65	28	56

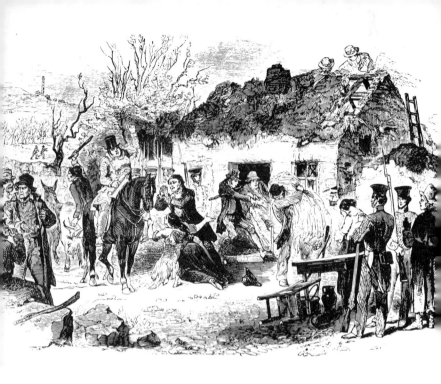

and pestilence it brought were complex. The laws governing the tenure of land by which the landlord possessed almost absolute power to evict his tenants and pull down their houses drove the farmers to go to almost any lengths to obtain money to pay their rents. Many did this by growing grain for sale and supporting themselves and their families almost exclusively on a diet of potatoes. This is not a matter of merely historical interest. In the West Indies, the principal crop is sugar, grown – not for the farmers to eat – but to be sold on the world market where its price is at the mercy of the blind and insensate laws of banking. Impoverished tropical nations grow cocoa, sisal, cotton or tobacco. There are good reasons why this is done. Nevertheless, a remote cause, for example, a technological development in the synthesis of 'man-made' fibres, or a change in fashion requiring Western women to be thin (and to give up chocolates) or for Western men to be healthy (and give up smoking) can initiate starvation in a remote nation half a world away.

8·2 'The ejectment of Irish Peasants', an engraving
from the *Illustrated London News* of 1848.
Landlords had absolute powers to evict
tenants. To pay their rent, many families were
forced to grow cereals for export and to live on any
potatoes that had survived the blight.

137

Another curious factor affecting the Irish famine of 1845 was the
sudden, unprecedented increase in the population which began in
the 1780s. At about this time the number of people in Ireland took
an abrupt upward leap. It is estimated that between 1779 and 1841
the population increased by more than 172 per cent. Today, when
it is customary to attribute our own population growth to improve-
ments in medical science, although close scrutiny shows that the
connection is by no means as simple as this, it is interesting to bear
the Irish increase in mind. So far, demography has failed to explain
it. Medical care in the country was derisory and industrialisation
with its accompanying accretion of wealth and activity had made
little or no impact.

But the most significant antecedent of the Irish famine was the
nature of the ecological environment in which the population subsisted. The biological species, man, in spite of its sophistication, its
education and self-awareness, is nevertheless, as are other species,
a creature that can only live within the balance of nature. And for
the Irish the balance, at first precarious, was finally upset. The
people living in poverty and resentment under a system of land
tenure in which whole communities could be turned off the farms
on which they had lived for centuries at a moment's notice became
dependent for food almost entirely on one single crop – the potato.

Potatoes were easy to grow in Ireland, they required very little
work beyond that needed for their sowing in the spring and digging
in the autumn and, above all, they could be saved for food if the
servants of the landlord or the soldiers supporting him came to
dispossess the farmer and destroy his house. Where other crops
could have been burned and destroyed, the subterranean potato,
only removable by hard work unacceptable alike to bailiffs and to
troops, remained. Every living organism lives in balance with its
environment. Animal populations are affected by other animal
species around them, by those they can see and fight – or flee – as
well as by micro-organisms which cannot be seen. Some of these
species, as well as the plant species, may serve as food. Climate and
weather, bringing plenty or scarcity, or encouraging one species at

the expense of another, also affect the situation even, on occasion, to the point of starvation.

The potato, like man, must also establish its balance in nature. In particular, potatoes grow in competition with the fungus *Phytophthora infestans*. This fungus, the potato blight, grows on the leaves of the plant. Spores, the seed of the fungus, are carried by wind or by raindrops, settle on the leaves where they send out mycelia, filamentous tubes, from which further spore-containing bodies develop. The zoospores when they develop, move throughout the plant, each in turn sending out further mycelial filaments and the entire potato plant is consumed. Furthermore, spores on an infected tuber may become transferred to sound potatoes in a store.

The life of the blight fungus is short. If the air is dry, the spore containers and the spores in them survive only for a few hours. In Ireland in 1845 and particularly in 1846, the weather conditions particularly favoured the spread of *Phytophthora infestans*. Throughout the summer of 1846 the weather was wet. On 6 June *The Times* recorded a heat wave, and yet at the same time it rained continuously. The origin of the potato blight fungus, like that of many other diseases, is obscure. A potato disease similar to blight was described in north Germany near Hanover in the 1830s and what was clearly blight caused a fully-recorded outbreak along the Atlantic coast of North America from Nova Scotia to Boston in 1842. It seems clear that the disease was endemic in the nineteenth century just as it is today, when constant precautions have to be taken by growers to ward off infection.

But although blight specifically due to *Phytophthora infestans* may not have been described before 1842, the potato crop was already known to be fickle before then. There had been a shortage in 1728 and again in 1739 and 1740. In the seasons of 1821 and 1822 failure in Munster and Connaught made it necessary for relief funds to be provided by the government. In all, twenty-four failures were listed by the Census of Ireland Commissioners of 1851. It followed, therefore, that in the fatal year of 1845 the un-

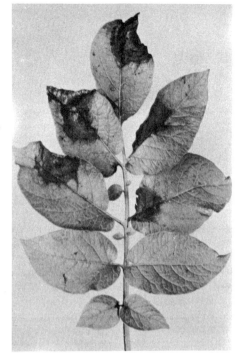

8·3 Potato blight caused by the fungus *Phytophthora infestans* on leaves and tubers.

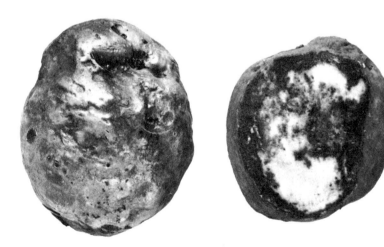

8·4 'From land to mouth.' Lord Boyd Orr, first Director-General of FAO ; a cartoon from the *Evening Standard* of 1946. It is not always a shortage of food that causes starvation ; sometimes it is a shortage of money.

reliability of the potato was accepted as an Act of God, like the vagaries of the weather. At the beginning of July of that year the weather was hot and dry and the crop promised well, then the weather suddenly changed and for upwards of three weeks there was 'one continuous gloom' with 'a succession of most chilling rain and some fog'. By September it was clear that blight had afflicted the potato crop. Over the country as a whole, the crop was not entirely lost but, like a patchwork quilt over the land, there were areas where not a sound potato was found. All became a stinking mass. Though hardship and short commons existed in many areas, they were not universal. Because some of the crop appeared healthy when dug but decayed later in store, a number of growers hurried to put their potatoes on the market so that in some areas supplies were unusually plentiful.

In 1846, however, every condition in the balance of nature favoured the spread of the blight fungus to an extent which had never existed before or has been recorded since. All biological species possess some ability to adjust themselves to unfavourable circumstances or to take advantage of favourable ones. Starvation is the ultimate failure of a species or community to cope with the circumstances of its environment, that is why it is an uncommon disaster rather than a continuing state of existence. The circumstances which combined in 1846 to produce a disastrous famine in Ireland during which men, women and children starved to death were various. The primary ones were biological: first, owing to the widespread dispersion of blight in 1845, many of the seed potatoes planted in 1846 were infected and the trash of the potato haulms left scattered over the fields also served to disperse the spores of the fungus widely; secondly, the long period of hot humid weather provided ideal conditions for their spread and proliferation. Besides these factors, there were social and cultural ones whose effects were equally significant. Such factors must always be borne in mind by students of food and nutrition. The dependence of the Irish on potatoes to the exclusion of almost every other staple food – a dependence arising, as I have already described, from Irish history –

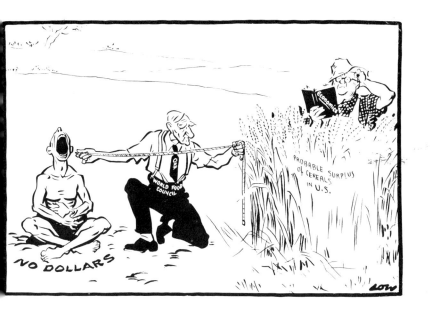

Text in image: PROBABLE SURPLUS OF CEREALS IN U.S. / WORLD FOOD COUNCIL / NO DOLLARS / LOW

was of cardinal significance. Then there were the laws of land tenure arising from which the landlord could – and did – evict his tenants from their farms and houses if they failed to grow and sell 'cash crops', principally cereal grains, to enable them to pay the rent. A modern nutritional scientist shows a lack of understanding of his subject if he believes that the *export* of food from Ireland, which continued throughout 1846 during the year of the most dreadful famine recorded in Europe in modern history, represented any particular circumstance or unusual hard-heartedness on the part of our ancestors. When presented with the estimate that, by the end of September in the year 1846, 60,000 tons of oats alone would have been exported, Sir Charles Trevelyan, the principal official at the Treasury in London insisted that such trade must not merely be permitted but encouraged on the grounds that only by following the economic principles of free trade would food, in the long run, flow into those places where it was most urgently needed. It must be recalled, as figure 8·4 shows, that the same principles produced very similar results a hundred years later when Sir John Boyd Orr, Director General of the Food and Agriculture Organisation of the United Nations, was attempting to avoid a similar state of affairs.

It is salutary to compare the onset of starvation, due to the mixture of climate, biological, social and political causes, in Ireland in 1845 with the starvation arising from the direct political action of cutting off the food supply to the Dutch in 1944. After the short artificial flush of plenty in the summer of 1845, when people quickly sold their potatoes for fear they should rot in store, a period of five or six months elapsed. By then in many areas every scrap of edible food had been eaten. In the spring of 1846, people were eating putrid potatoes and dysentery was widespread. The Government issued small supplies of maize, which had been bought as a relief measure, but would only sanction its issue to men who could pay for it with wages earned by working at public projects or who were inmates of a 'workhouse'. The old, the sick, women and children were excluded; economic doctrine taught that only when food prices were high did adequate supplies flow into the districts where they were needed. On 31 August 1846, in Westport in County Mayo, where by then conditions were reported to be 'indescribable' and 'a nest of fever and vermin', hunger drove a 'large and orderly body of people' to march to Westport House to appeal for help to Lord Sligo. When he came out, someone cried, 'Kneel, kneel!' and the crowd dropped on its knees before him.

By 25 September – this was 1846 when, after the serious but partial failure of the potato crop in 1845, the entire crop for the second season had been lost – people were living on blackberries in County Waterford and on cabbage leaves in County Cork. But in the parish of Cloone, with 22,000 inhabitants, people were reported to be starving by hundreds.

By the winter of 1846, the classical social picture of starvation was established. The poorer members of the population, those who normally lived as 'squatters' in huts built of sods cut from the bog and subsisted on the potatoes they grew, abandoned their hovels and descended on the towns in droves. In the words of an eye-witness, a Father Mathew, these unhappy beings 'slept in ditches and in doorways, begged, and were driven away and, in Cork alone died at the rate of one hundred a week.' In County Clare, an Inspecting Officer wrote of 'women and little children, crowds of

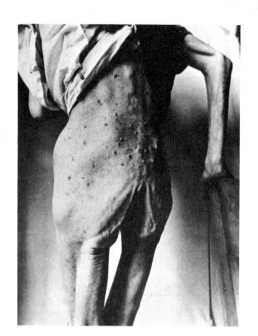

8·5 Lack of flesh and muscle, with dry parchment-like skin, are typical signs of starvation.

whom were to be seen scattered over the turnip fields like a flock of famished crows, devouring the raw turnips, mothers half naked, shivering in the snow and sleet, uttering exclamations of despair while their children were screaming with hunger.' Another observer, writing of conditions in the village of Skibbereen, described entering a hovel in which 'six famished and ghastly skeletons, to all appearance dead, were huddled in a corner on some filthy straw . . . their wretched legs hanging about, naked above the knees'. But perhaps the most explicit and accurate description was that of Sidney Godolphin Osborne of conditions in Donegal in the spring of 1847: 'Attenuation seems to have absorbed all appearance of flesh or muscle', skin was rough and dry like parchment and hung in folds, eyes were sunken, the shoulder-bones were so high that the neck seemed to have sunk into the chest, face and neck were so wasted as to look like a skull, the hair was thin and all had a pallor such as Osborne had never seen before.

He described the children as suffering most: they were skeletons, the skin over their chest, bones and abdomen stretched so tight that every curve of their breast bone and ribs stood out in relief.

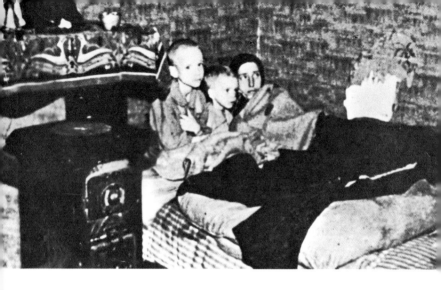

'No words can describe the appearance of the arms', he wrote, 'from below the elbow the two bones seem to be stripped of every atom of flesh. If you take hold of the loose skin within the elbow joint, and lift the arm by it, it comes away in a long, thin fold as if you had lifted one side of a long narrow bag in which some bones had been placed'.

Osborne acutely observed and wrote of the terrible circumstances of real starvation of which nutritionists read today in the cold pages of scientific textbooks. He saw starving children approaching their end: 'In the very act of death still not a tear nor a cry,' he wrote, 'I have scarcely ever seen one try to change his or her position . . . two, three or four in a bed, there they lie and die, if suffering still ever silent, unmoved'. By April 1847, children were looking like little old men and women of eighty years of age, wrinkled and bent and, most horrible of all, the hair on their heads had fallen out and, instead, hair grew on their faces. A Quaker, Mr R.D. Webb, reported that starving Irish children 'look like monkeys'. In modern scientific research, starvation has been observed to affect the endocrine glands. This is thought to be due to the disturbance of protein metabolism. The hormones produced by the endocrine glands are chemical combinations of protein and it is therefore to be expected that under conditions of extreme protein deficiency, the production of hormones will be disturbed. Amenorrhoea and delayed puberty are common features in starving women and girls. Men lose their libido and become impotent; sometimes their breasts develop. And in children, as with other non-nutritional endocrine disturbances, there may be this strange growth of so-called 'lanugo' hair.

Foods can be described in terms of their chemical composition and nutrition can be studied from the point of view of the biochemical functions of the separate nutrients of which the diet is composed. Starvation can be investigated in just such a manner and, indeed, Professor Ancel Keys at the University of Minnesota conducted in 1950 a classical investigation on a number of volunteers which enabled him and his collaborators to publish a book, *The Biology of Human Starvation*, which constituted a milestone in nutritional understanding. This is one way, and an important way, to advance knowledge. Nevertheless, starvation – like other nutritional conditions – is also a social phenomenon and for that reason its effects and causes under 'field' conditions must also be observed by those who purport to possess a proper understanding of the subject.

Students of nutrition, while taking note of the loss of weight and the emaciation of starvation, of hunger oedema and the effect of famine on the mental condition, should also take note of the fact that even during the terrible winter of 1847–8 an observer, Richard Milnes, who came to Ireland to assess the state of people in the famine areas, stayed at several country houses where he found life going on as usual. At the seat of the Marquess of Headfort in County Meath, there was a party and charades in the evening. The guests staying in Kilkenny with Lord Bessborough, a man noted for his kindness to his tenants, hunted all day and engaged in amateur dramatics at night. In Dublin in the spring of 1847 when labourers were being discharged from public works in tens of thousands and had barely enough food to keep themselves alive, when typhus had broken out and was raging in the town, the social season for the fashionable well-to-do people, always noted for its gaiety, was as lively as ever.

The famine and the starvation which it caused in north west Holland in the Second World War began with the stoppage of food supplies in 1944 and ended with their restoration in 1945. The community suffered and many of the people died. But when relief came the sufferers and the community of which they were a part were restored to health. The famine in Ireland afflicted a community already socially sick. In 1845 when the potato crop failed in part, the people were poor, unhappy, disorganised and ignorant. The famine continued through 1846, when the entire potato crop, almost the sole source of food, was lost, and through 1847 when the people had been too weak and despairing to plant a proper crop, even when the seed potatoes had not themselves been used for food. Towards its end, famine was made more horrible still by fever. When it was over, not only had this nutritional disaster destroyed people, it had also destroyed the Irish community. Thousands of those families who survived took ship from their devastated country to America and Canada where, having brought the fever with them, many of them died before they could set foot ashore in the quarantine stations on Grosse Isle in the St Lawrence river or in the immigrant sheds in Montreal.

Starvation is a distinct state due to so severe a lack of food that, if the state continues, the patient dies. Starvation produces signs and symptoms by which it can be recognised. It is, therefore, seriously misleading to make careless estimates of the total number of people in a community – or in the world as a whole – who are 'starving'. On the other hand, even when some people are in fact starving, it does not follow that the whole population of which they are members is suffering. It may be equally misleading to visit the Holland of 1945–6 or, for that matter, the United States of 1968 and assume, at a glance, that nobody is starving in either place.

9 Social behaviour and economics

There are many lessons to be learned from the Irish famine of 1845–7 which has been discussed in chapter 8. One of the more important is that, although the nutritional disaster which caused the death of one and a half million people was primarily due to a shortage of calories, that is to say, to lack of food, it can be argued that it was equally due to poverty, in other words to lack of money, and, of course, to reliance on a single food crop. It is well recognised by nutritionists that underfeeding and malnutrition may occur within nations plentifully provided with food if the food supplies are unequally distributed. And poverty is by far the most important factor responsible for unequal distribution. It does the starving beggar little good to tell him that the dining room of the Ritz Hotel accepts all customers without discrimination when he has no money to pay for a meal.

In 1935, Sir John Boyd Orr, as he then was, studied the diet of 1,152 working-class families distributed throughout Great Britain. He also collected information about their incomes and, after having surveyed in detail the food consumed by each family for a week, he calculated the nutritional value of their diet and then compared the intake of nutrients with the estimated nutritional requirements of the individual members of the families. The results of this work were published in what is now a classic of its kind entitled *Food, Health and Income*. Orr estimated that the lowest economic group comprising 10 per cent of the population, representative of four and a half million people were living on a diet which failed to provide enough calories, protein, vitamin A, vitamin C, iron and calcium to reach the level required for proper nutrition. In the next two economic groups, the families of semi-skilled workers, small shop-keepers and the like, covering 40 per cent of the population, although they were eating enough in terms of calories and protein, intake of vitamins and minerals was below standard. Orr's survey showed in quantitative terms not only what everybody knew, that poorer people ate a less varied and plentiful diet than richer people, but that the diet of the less well-to-do in Great Britain in the 1930s was of unsatisfactory nutritional composition.

9·1 School children in 1894 (*top*) and at the same school in 1944 (*bottom*). In 50 years, prosperity brought a change in buildings, in clothes, in cheerfulness, and in nutrition.

Orr in his survey related the amount of money which people had to spend to the nutritional adequacy of the diet they ate. Adequacy was assessed by comparing the calorific value of the total food supply and its content of nutrients with the estimated requirements for health. It was not possible in this survey to study the health of the members of the actual families whose weekly food consumption was measured nor to determine whether they showed any of the recognisable signs and symptoms of one or other of the deficiency states known to arise from malnutrition. The circumstantial evidence which he presented was, however, strong. In any event, so closely are the various social factors interlocked that the specific contribution of nutritional inadequacy is more frequently than not difficult to disentangle from that arising from other causes.

Poverty brings many ills; poverty is commonly associated with an inadequate diet and sometimes, as was done by Sir John Boyd Orr, the precise inadequacy can be calculated in terms of kilocalories, protein, vitamins and minerals; poverty is frequently accompanied by poor health. Although it is not always easy to prove that the nutritional deficiency was the direct cause of the ill health – after all, it might also be caused by poor housing, overcrowding, inadequate clothing or arduous and unhealthy work – it is reasonable to assume that it plays a part.

Between 1923 and 1927, McGonigle and Kirby studied the state of health of a group of people, largely made up of poorly paid industrial workers, living in a particular slum area of the English town of Stockton-on-Tees. Whereas in Stockton-on-Tees as a whole the so-called 'standardised quinquennial death-rate' was 12 per 10,000 of the population, in two separate parts of the slum area it was 23 and 26 per 10,000. In 1927, part of the slum area was pulled down and a modern housing estate providing greatly superior housing and sanitary conditions erected in its place. McGonigle and Kirby then collected the mortality statistics for the years 1928–32. They found that, far from having improved the state of health of the people, as measured in terms of the mortality figures, the improved housing had worsened the situation. The

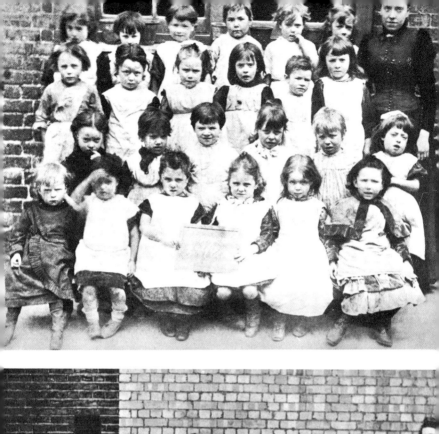
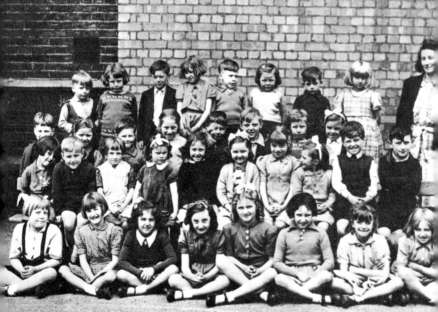

death rate of the rehoused community had increased to 34 per 10,000, whereas that of a comparable group who had continued to live in the remaining slum houses that had not been pulled down, had remained at 23 per 10,000. The only explanation provided by McGonigle and Kirby for this state of affairs was that the higher rents of the new houses reduced the amount of money available for food to the people living in them by 11d. per head per week and that it was this exacerbation of their poverty and malnutrition that was reflected in their higher rate of mortality.

The relationship between money, diet and health was demonstrated in a more direct way in the life's work of Seebohm Rowntree. Between 1899 and 1950 he studied the incomes of working-class families in the city of York, he recorded the amount of food they were able to buy and, in the light of the gradually increasing understanding of nutritional science during the period of his work, assessed its nutritional adequacy and, finally, he collected statistics about their health.

The basis of Rowntree's approach was to calculate what he termed the 'poverty line'. This was the minimum amount of money needed by a family, made up of a man, his wife and three children, to buy at the lowest cost a diet which would just support satisfactory nutrition. This concept enabled him to divide the families in York into various groups and study these groups separately. As an example of the results he obtained, we may usefully consider the 1936 survey. There was then a group, A/B, whose income brought them below the 'poverty line'. Rowntree, like other investigators both before his time and since, was not able to pick out specific indications of malnutrition (and he forebore to talk loosely, as is sometimes done today, of 'starvation') but he was able to collect what are perhaps the two most direct general indications of the health of a community, that is, the standardised death rate and the number of babies dying in their first year (the infant mortality rate). Among the group A/B, whose lack of money held them below the 'poverty line', the standardised death rate was 13·5 and the infant mortality rate was 77·7 per 1,000 live births. In contrast to these figures, he found for the D/E group, who had incomes bringing them above the 'poverty line', a standardised death rate of 8·4 and an infant mortality rate of 41·3 per 1,000 live births.

Although the information available to Rowntree at the time did not enable him to do so, it is now possible to calculate from his records the nutritional composition of the diets eaten by the A/B and the D/E groups. The consumption of animal protein was 25 g per 'man' among the A/Bs compared with 42 g per 'man' among the D/Es. And while the amount of vitamin A eaten by the D/Es exceeded their estimated requirements, the A/Bs were only obtaining 52 per cent of what they needed as a fully adequate intake.

Here then in the same population we have facts which can reasonably be interpreted to show that the money income which a family has available may be reflected in terms of kilocalories, protein and vitamin A. Rowntree not only showed this for a particular survey, done at a particular time. He was also able to show that in 1899, that is thirty-seven years earlier when people in York were relatively poorer and when the diet eaten by A/Bs was even more unsatisfactory in nutritional terms, their death rate was 27·6, not 13·5 as it became in 1936, and of each 1,000 babies born alive 247, not 77·7, died before their first birthday. And in 1899, the D/Es, whose income brought them above the 'poverty line', had a mortality of 13·5 and an infant mortality rate of 173 per 1,000 live births. Hence, although social medicine as a whole was less advanced and life was harder in 1899 than in 1936, those with more money still obtained a better diet (this, after all, was Rowntree's definition of 'poverty line') and their mortality statistics were better too. The same picture was repeated in 1950 when Rowntree completed, after half a century, his third study of conditions in York.

Scientific knowledge about food composition combined with nutritional knowledge about the physiological needs of different types of people, of men doing sedentary work or engaged in heavy labour, of expectant mothers, children and adolescents, make it possible to draw up a table showing the composition of a nutritionally adequate diet. This problem is solved. A problem which is

9·2 Bonteheuwel, near Cape Town in South Africa, one of the Cape-coloured settlements for families of mixed racial origin, where the income of the family was found to reflect the degree of infantile diarrhoea and the state of nutrition.

not solved, however, is how best a community whose diet is inadequate can provide themselves with a nutritionally adequate one.

I have written that the problem is how malnourished people 'can provide themselves' with a better diet. At the present time, many people and organisations among the more fortunate communities of the world have felt themselves moved to try to provide help for those in less prosperous circumstances. Elaborate schemes of 'welfare' have been organised, charitable organisations have donated dried milk and vitamins, nutritional and agricultural experts have visited the so-called 'developing' nations. These experts have achieved much but the problem has not been solved. After a generation of welfare schemes by which the richer nations designed to provide help, the gap separating them from those whose nutrition they wish to improve has become wider rather than narrower.

There are many reasons why this is so. It has been said that 'he who provides a poor man with a fish satisfies his hunger for a day but he who teaches the poor man how to catch fish for himself provides him with food for the rest of his life'. Gifts of food undoubtedly do good, yet they often do less good than was intended. The food may be different from that to which the recipients are accustomed and part will consequently be wasted. Or again, relief supplies may never reach those for whom they were intended but may instead be sold for profit by the middlemen responsible for their distribution.

In chapter 8, writing of the Irish famine of 1845–7, I described the devotion of the Government to the economic beliefs of the time that it would be both unwise and morally wrong to issue relief supplies of maize to replace the blighted potatoes free or at a price cheaper than that currently prevailing on the market. More than a century later it has come to be believed that relief food supplies should be not merely cheaper than the market rate but may even be issued free. It may perhaps come about that when this policy is, in its turn, examined dispassionately in the future it may be seen to

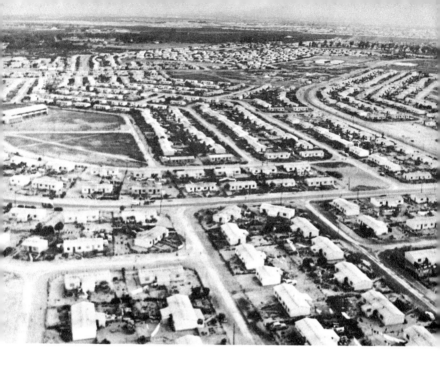

be equally as mistaken as that of the nineteenth century admini-strators of Ireland. There is, indeed, much evidence to support the proposition that the provision of money is a better and more direct way of treating malnutrition than the provision of food, or rather, that to enable malnourished people to earn sufficient money is the best way of all.

Consider the recent survey carried out in South Africa (Wittmann, W., Moodie, A.D., Fellingham, S.A. and Hansen, J.D.L., *S. Afric Med.* J., 41, 664, 1967). A study was made of a group of so-called 'Cape Coloured' families of mixed racial origin. These people were living in solidly built houses with tiled floors, asbestos roofs, electricity and piped water. The investigation covered the food consumption of the people, their health and nutritional condition and their income and social status. When all the families studied were divided into four groups, according to the amount of weekly income remaining after rent had been paid divided by the number of persons in the household, the following facts emerged.

From each of the four groups, 30 children under four years of age were chosen at random and visited every two weeks for a year. First of all it was found that the average height and weight of the children from the poorest group were lowest and the averages for all four groups fell into order according to income. This was taken as an indication that the poorest children were not getting enough to eat and also were not eating enough protein. The lack of protein was verified by the determination of albumen levels in their blood serum. But the most striking difference between the wellbeing of the four groups was in the incidence and severity of diarrhoea among the groups of young children. Almost three quarters of those coming from the poorest group suffered severely from diarrhoea at some time during the year's investigation and almost half had repeated attacks. There were altogether 100 episodes of diarrhoea among the 30 children of the poorest group, and fewer and fewer in the second and third best off, while in the group with the most money to spend only 25 outbreaks occurred.

The lesson for the nutritional scientist is one that it is important for him or her to learn. It is that shortage of money is not only associated with shortage of food but also with the dirt and consequent infection of poor home circumstances. For example, lice were found most frequently in the poorest group of households. The South African research workers reached the conclusion that poverty and the consequent inadequate provision of food and particularly the relative shortage of meat, eggs and milk causes malnutrition which itself is conducive to diarrhoea in the young children of the household which is exacerbated by poor housekeeping, dirt and overcrowding. The signs and symptoms of malnutrition so crisply described in the scientific textbooks do not occur by themselves but are often only part of the confused mixture of deficiency symptoms, infection and squalor compounded of poverty. At least, Dr Wittmann and his colleagues, assessing the results of their study, strongly argue that, rather than instruction in hygiene and nutrition or the institution of welfare schemes, which the poorest people often fail to understand, an increased family income – that is money – is the best treatment.

Nobody *wants* to be malnourished and yet there are few people for whom the consumption of a nutritionally perfect diet ranks especially high in their scale of social priorities. Even people who are sufficiently educated to know that an excessive consumption of sugar is bad and that a regular consumption of fruit and vegetables is good can be found nevertheless eating sugar and neglecting to eat vegetables and fruit. The fact is that people behave in this way, whether they are well-to-do business-men or poor members of an impoverished community. In a series of studies carried out in Toronto in Canada, it was found that a large number of families were eating insufficient calcium and thiamine (vitamin B_1) for their needs. These people were advised by the nutritional scientists that they could remedy these defects in their diet – and without adding to the cost – if they would only buy and eat dried skim-milk powder in place of some of the sweet cakes, fried potatoes and canned soup on which they chose to spend their money. They were also advised to eat whole-meal bread in place of the white bread they preferred and – in order specifically to increase the thiamine content of the diet – to make a point of eating more lean pork. To increase the ascorbic acid (vitamin C) content of their diet, the poorest families were advised to buy oranges and grapefruit even if it put up the cost of their food.

Such advice may be useful; on the other hand, its usefulness is limited because the motive to eat a better and healthier diet is only one among a number of the motives by which human behaviour is controlled, and it may not be the strongest.

In the winter of 1945, the citizens of Vienna in Austria were suffering considerable hardship. The situation was far short of famine but food was scarce. World War II had come to an end in Europe but the normal supply routes to the city were disrupted and food supplies were being brought in with some difficulty through the port of Trieste. The city itself was divided up into six sections, one administered by the Americans, one by the Russians, one by the French, two subsections by the British and the centre by a con-sortium of all four powers. A rationing system was in operation

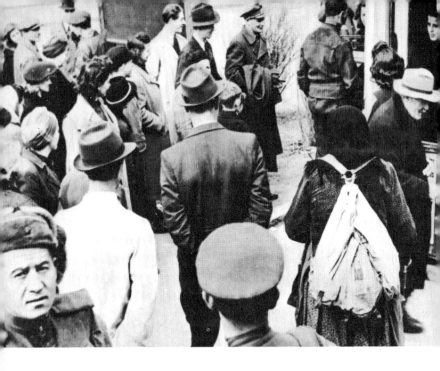

but the amount of food available was barely sufficient for maintenance. It consequently happened, as always happens under such circumstances, that the poorest and most defenceless members of the community suffered from malnutrition. In order to deal with the situation, the administering authorities set up welfare systems with a view to mitigating the most serious effects of the food shortage. It is, I think, instructive to compare the two contrasting approaches to this same problem followed by the American and by the British welfare services in Vienna at the time.

The people in the American sector of the city who applied for assistance, after having their credentials properly checked and their family circumstances documented, were then examined one by one, were weighed and measured and then moved in line, first to a table where they were given a vitamin tablet to swallow, next, if it was appropriate to their case, they were given a tablet containing iron, or calcium or halibut-liver oil, or a glass of reconstituted dried milk. In the main, those receiving aid were old, or were women with their children. And each one was given the dietary supplement best cal-

9·3 A street-weighing scene in Vienna in March 1946. When food is scarce people do not suffer equally. Those who are really getting too little can be identified by their loss in weight.

157

culated to make good the nutritional deficiencies from which he or she was suffering.

The principle followed by the British medical authorities was different. Families deemed to be specially in need, their need having been assessed so far as was possible from an inspection of their domestic circumstances, sent one member to the administrative depot where each was given a food parcel. The parcel contained a mixture of what was available: condensed milk, canned meat, flour, sugar, cooking fat. The selection of foods was chosen to supply the specific nutrients known to be needed, so far as this could be done, according to the needs of the people concerned. Hence, in so far as they ate the food, their nutritional state was benefited. But often, the woman of the family did not eat the food herself; instead she gave it to her husband. And sometimes she sold part of it and spent the money on clothes or bedding, or to repair the house – or perhaps on cigarettes.

The biblical statement that 'man doth not live by bread only, but by every word that proceedeth out of the mouth of the Lord doth man live' applies as directly to the present situation of the scientific and technological period of history as it did to the situation existing when it was written. It is important therefore for food scientists to make as much effort to understand the beliefs and motives of the community with which they are concerned as they do to assess the nutritional composition of the food supplies which make up their diet. Just as it is found that only rarely does it happen that a single deficiency, say, of vitamin C or niacin, exists leading to clearly defined scurvy or pellagra, but instead there is a mixed deficiency of several nutrients, often complicated by infection and exposure, so also must it be recognised that all these may, in a real human situation, also be further enmeshed in strains arising from the need to pay rent, educate children, travel long distances to work, flee from enemies, or provide a dowry either in money or goods. But while it is possible to draw up a schedule, showing in quantitative terms the needs for a list of different food constituents, such as that shown in table 6·3, it is not possible to make a balance-sheet of the diverse social pressures to which men and women are exposed, even though those are equally important. An orthodox Jew would die of hunger rather than eat pork, just as a devout Hindu would starve rather than eat beef. Most curious of all, perhaps, is the fact that a Christian, even one with a scientific education, who would readily accept a transfusion of human blood, or the transplant of a dead man's heart, would perish rather than eat the flesh of a corpse.

We can recognise our own strong feelings about the beliefs under-lying the behaviour of our own society, whether they be the need to pay rent or alternatively the provision of housing as a welfare service, which can be construed as a direct contribution to nutri-tion, or ideas about foods which it is appropriate for us to eat or, on the contrary, which we consider disgusting. Nutritional workers and food scientists working outside their own countries must, therefore, be prepared to recognise, even if they do not share, the equally strong feelings of other societies. For example, a team of scientists observed that the diet of certain groups in the Chin States of Upper Burma was seriously deficient in animal protein. After considerable study a way was found to improve the situation by cross-breeding the small local breed of black pigs which were raised by the farmers with an improved strain to obtain progeny giving a greater yield of meat. The entire operation, however, com-pletely failed to benefit the nutrition of the population because of one fact which had been overlooked as irrelevant. The cross-bred pigs were spotted. And it was firmly believed – as firmly as we believe that to eat, say, mice, would be disgusting – that spotted pigs were unfit to eat.

Dr M. M. Autret, head of the Nutrition Division of the Food and Agriculture Organisation of the United Nations, reported in 1962 a similar incident. This was the introduction into a certain area of sorghum (millet) as a cereal crop to provide food at a time of the year when alternative supplies were scarce. The local population, however, refused to eat it; it was their firm belief that sorghum was only suitable for donkeys. In reflecting on this incident, it is perhaps pertinent to recall that in the eighteenth century Dr Samuel

9·4 Taboo animals. Even hungry people do not eat everything that is eatable. Large numbers of people in different parts of the world would rather die than eat such 'disgusting' creatures as horses, oxen, chickens, dogs, camels or pigs.

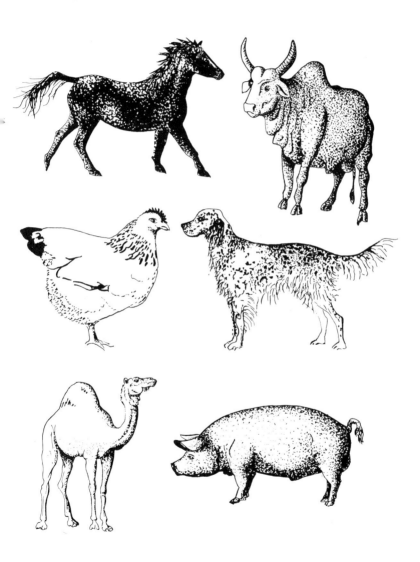

Johnson in writing his English dictionary defined oats as, 'a grain, which in England is generally given to horses, but in Scotland supports the people'.

The science of nutrition can, in one sense, be considered to be a branch of physiology. That is to say, an unconscious man brought into hospital with severe brain damage after a traffic accident can be kept alive for many months by intravenous injections of a sterile mixture of glucose (to provide kilocalories), amino acids, minerals and vitamins. On the other hand, nutrition can equally be taken to be one of the aspects of anthropology, the science of human behaviour. And food habits are one factor of it. A giant panda in a zoo has nutritional requirements, just as a man has, and those requirements can be expressed in terms of vitamins and protein and the other necessary food components. But if the panda does not receive its nutrients in the form of bamboo shoots, it will die. People, being more rational than animals, can be made to change their customs, but customs are important attributes of their well-being nevertheless. Professor Stoetzel, of the Sorbonne in Paris, has pointed out the significance of food habits. Studies in France of the behaviour of Jewish immigrants from Tunisia showed that they could quite readily be persuaded to change their language and that, in due course, many of them changed their religion. But it was also found that both these changes took place before they changed their food habits. This aspect of their behaviour was deeply rooted.

A more subtle example of the way in which dietary prejudices, which have no recognisable basis of nutritional logic, can nevertheless affect the nutritional value of diet is shown in the eating habits of British coal miners. These men, because of the nature of their work, carry a meal with them to eat mid-way through their shift. During the course of a survey it was found that not only did the amount they ate, as measured in terms of kilocalories, vary very widely but that the amount of cheese included in the mid-shift meal varied from district to district almost ten-fold. This variation was based on a firmly held belief in the areas where little or no cheese was eaten in the mine, that its consumption was positively harmful.

Table 9·1 Comparison of the calorific value of the food eaten underground by coal miners in different parts of Britain

Coalfield	Average energy value of mid-shift meal	Proportion of day's requirement	Average daily cheese consumption
	(Kilocalories)	(%)	(oz)
Leicestershire	1,100	28	1·9
South Wales	1,100	28	1·8
Fifeshire	950	24	1·1
Yorkshire	840	22	0·9
Lancashire	650	17	0·2
Durham	610	16	0·2

Figures are shown in table 9·1.

Food habits are very firmly fixed. They can, however, be changed although change may not be easily brought about. For example, the coal miners in Durham, as a population group, were, at the time the survey to which I have referred was carried out, firmly convinced that to eat cheese when working in the pit was harmful. Nevertheless, it was also observed that when a Durham miner moved from his own district and went to work in Scotland, he fairly quickly changed his habits and in due course was found to be prepared to eat as much cheese as a Scottish miner.

But although food habits can be changed, it is important for nutritional scientists to be aware that they exist and, if possible, to have some understanding of their origin. The scientist can never afford to take them lightly. Ignorance of dietary customs and food habits may lead to disaster, and not only to nutritional disaster. It can be recalled that the Indian Mutiny against the rule of the British in India in 1857, which cost many lives and caused suffering and distress throughout the sub-continent, was initiated by the horror of the Indian troops at the idea of eating beef and at the possibility that a rumour – it was no more than this – might be true that the rifle bullets with which they had been issued had been greased with beef fat.

Professor Frederick Simoons, in his scholarly monograph on the basis of the main food customs and beliefs throughout the world, has pointed out that the problem of providing food for the diverse communities of which the world population is made up is only partly one of improving agricultural methods and the techniques of food manufacture, and is only partly a matter of coping with the rising numbers of people in the different countries of the world. The other side of the problem of equal importance is the nature of the customs of these different peoples. Simoons examined the cultural and religious beliefs against the eating of beef, chickens, eggs and pork by one group of communities, and against the consumption of dog flesh, camel flesh and horse flesh by another set of peoples.

These prejudices derive from very deep roots, some of which are quite extraordinary and all of which are irrational, The antipathy of Anglo-Saxon nations to the eating of horse meat is merely one example. In nutritional terms, horse meat is an excellent food. The amino acid composition of its proteins makes it well suited to human nutrition. It contains a higher concentration of glycogen than most other meat and tends, consequently, to keep well. Furthermore, the horse suffers from few diseases capable of harming man and possesses singularly hygienic habits. Horse meat is widely consumed in wide areas of Asia from the borders of Eastern Europe to Mongolia. The prejudice against it in those countries in which it is taboo apparently became fixed subsequent to the year A D 732 when Pope Gregory III ordered Boniface, the apostle to the Germans, to forbid the eating of horse flesh in order that those who were Christians could be seen to be different from the pagans among whom they lived and for whom horse meat was a common article of diet.

The prejudice against eating the flesh of pigs appears to be of even greater antiquity. There are peoples scattered widely throughout the world who eat pork and there is good archaeological evidence to show that pigs, together with dogs, were among the first animals to be domesticated by man. Both species were kept partly as scavengers but also for use as food. Yet in the Middle East, parts of

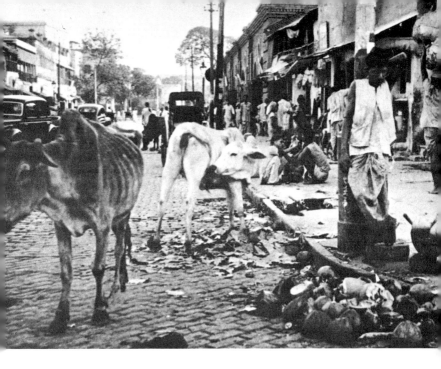

Asia including areas of India, and in several parts of Africa, the eating of pig-meat is taboo. This avoidance, like most other dietary prejudices, appears to be completely irrational and has no nutritional basis. The proposition that the Jews rejected pork because it was particularly perishable would not have prevented its immediate use for feasts. If, however, the objection is argued to be the pig's habit of scavenging, why were not poultry similarly proscribed? It has more recently been suggested that pork was avoided because it can be a source of the disease *trichinosis*, due to the presence in it of the parasitic worm *Trichinella spiralis*. Although this infection is known to be a hazard at the present day and makes it dangerous to eat pork or food, such as sausages containing pork, uncooked (cooking destroys the parasite), this could certainly not have been known in pre-scientific times. The time-lapse between infection and the appearance of the disease is so great that the significance of uncooked pork as the cause of trichinosis was only discovered comparatively recently.

To those people who think of nutritional health in terms of

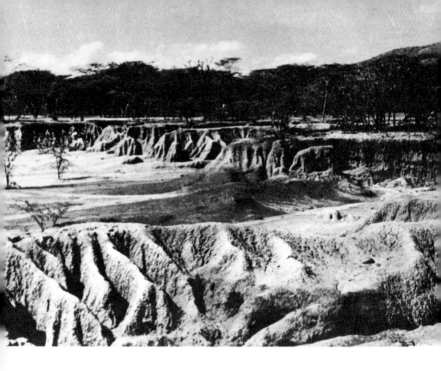

calories and protein and diet as measured by the consumption of meat, dairy products, fruit, vegetables and cereals, either in the unprocessed condition or after having been processed and packaged by one or other of the sophisticated procedures of modern technology, the effect of the beliefs and idiosyncrasies of tribal behaviour appear to be nothing more than a troublesome aberration. It is common for those educated in terms of modern scientific technology, who sincerely hold the welfare of developing nations at heart, to be impatient at the religious beliefs of Hindus who, feeling that life – even the life of animals – is sacred, refuse to kill cattle for food. By this belief it can be seen all too easily that India, a country containing a third of the world's total population of cattle, yet a country poor and overpopulated, deprives its people of badly needed food. This is true; and there is a certain blunt simplicity in the direct 'scientific' approach inherent in the proposition that the Indians ought to issue contraceptive pills to their women and slaughter their sacred cows for food.

Yet, as I have said before, anthropology is a science as well as

9·6 Soil erosion in Kenya. Overstocking causes loss of plant cover so that rain water flows too rapidly over the ground and produces gulleys.

165

nutrition. And if Hindus have beliefs by which they guide their behaviour and influence their nutrition so also have Western scientists. The settlers in North America believing, as do the generality of Western peoples, that all the creatures and plants on earth are there for the use of man, exterminated the buffaloes, ploughed up the prairies and, within a generation, had created a 'dust-bowl'. We, in our generation in the pursuit of fat for the manufacture of margarine and, unlike the Hindus, careless of the life of animals, have all but exterminated the largest creature on earth, the whale.

Part 3

Food technology, present and future

10 The evolution of technological processes

Perhaps the most striking effect of the application of science and of technology based on science to the affairs of modern society has been the rapid urbanisation of a major part of the world's population. Whereas in 1800, only 25 per cent of the population of England and Wales lived in cities of 100,000 people or more, by 1900, when the country had become industrialised, 76 per cent of the population lived in large towns. The same phenomenon overtook countries which embraced the ideas of technology later than the English. In the great territories of the United States, it was 1875 before 25 per cent of the people lived in large towns; by 1950, the proportion was 65 per cent. Japan, the first nation in Asia to accept industrialisation, saw the proportion of Japanese who lived in towns rise from 22 per cent in 1925 to 60 per cent in 1960. And the same change has occurred and continues throughout the world.

Whereas people who live in the country and subsist by farming depend for their sustenance on agriculture, to feed the town-dweller, and particularly to supply the great cities which continuously increase in size, the resources of food technology are needed. The trend towards urbanisation which removes people from the sources of food supply has stimulated the development of foods and food products which can be shipped long distances and, as is necessary for the orderly distribution for the great numbers which constitute our modern cities, can be stored for many months. This necessity for stability however, presents certain difficulties, the solution of which, either in whole or in part, has stimulated some of the more remarkable of the scientific developments in food processing. For example, to prepare flour so that it will keep without deteriorating, it is essential to separate not only the outer husk, but also the embryo and its associated structures. The effect of this is, as is shown in figure 10·1, to remove much of the vitamin content. Similarly, prolonged storage and the processes of freezing, canning and dehydration of fruits, vegetables, meats and dairy products may also involve loss of nutrients before the food reaches the urban population for whom it is intended.

But just as modern technology has been developed with remarkable success to preserve food – by freezing, drying, canning, the use of preservatives ranging from wood-smoke and hops to the modern chemical additives provided by chemical science, and by other means – so also can this same scientific understanding provide the knowledge by which any nutrients which may be lost can be replaced. Similarly, although processed foods taste good and are often of excellent consistency, sometimes their flavour and consistency are not *quite* so good as those of fresh food harvested and distributed in prime condition. Much of the efforts of food scientists and technologists working in the laboratories of the great food firms are today spent in attempts to achieve what might be considered to be trivial aesthetic ends, such as to make dried milk powder more compact so that a unit weight can be packed in a smaller, cheaper container, or to make a powder which will recombine with water more quickly. Intense efforts are being devoted to the study of taste and smell; and an equal investment of the time of trained scientists and technologists is devoted to the study of the consistency of food. As I describe below, study is even made of the noise produced by processed foods when they are bitten. It is accepted that this characteristic is of significance in assessing the quality of such articles as biscuits (crackers), celery and prepared breakfast cereals.

But apart from these peripheral attributes of food technology – peripheral but nevertheless important, as the last chapter makes plain – the fundamental importance of modern food technology is as an essential means of rendering food, which by its very nature is subject to deterioration and decay, stable.

In 1961, L. A. W. Howard, of the West African Stored Products Research Unit, which was part of the Federal Ministry of Commerce and Industry in Lagos, Nigeria, published a report of a survey of losses of quality, and of food, sustained during the transport of dried fish obtained from Lake Chad and adjoining rivers before it reached its market. The fish caught in Lake Chad in Central Africa and in the rivers nearby is processed by primitive methods. Two main techniques are used. Some types of fish, notably *Alestes* and

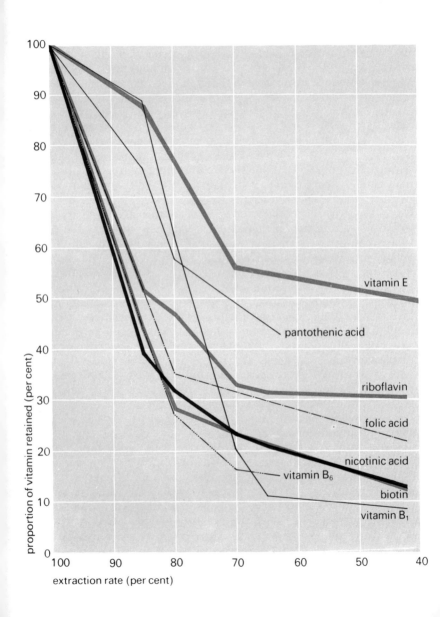

10·1 Relation between the milling extraction rate and the proportion of the total vitamins in the grain retained in the flour.

Tilapia, are dried whole, others are cut in half and dried in a kiln over a smoky fire. Alternatively the fish may be partly charred on a fire of burning grass or smoked and partly roasted on a grid. These processes may all be combined with some measure of sun-drying or, in some places, the whole drying process may be done in the sun. After from three to six days the process is considered to be finished and the dried fish, now called 'banda' is ready for dispatch to the market.

Just as the processing of this fish is done without the use of any of the methods of modern food technology, so also is its means of transport – at least for part of its journey to market – equally lacking in modernity. The dried fish is collected from the fishermen in bales or sacks and is transported along bush tracks on the back of a camel, a donkey, or an ox. Much of the fish, transported in this way, is carried to an entrepot market at Maiduguri. After having been unloaded there, perhaps unpacked and then repacked, the fish passes on its way to the ultimate consumer in Lagos, or through Jos in the eastern region.

When the fish is first caught and while it is being got ready for drying in the villages where the fishermen live, it attracts flies of several species which lay their eggs in it. If it is smoked or charred immediately it is caught, a hard dry surface is produced which resists the attack of these flies. With few exceptions, however, all such dried fish is liable to be attacked by *Dermestids*. In addition, the dried fish, even though its smoked pellicle resists fly infestation, has cracks and fissures leaving the internal moist parts exposed and liable to extensive damage. The fish dried only in the sun is most susceptible of all and the infestation was found to reach an extraordinary level. It can be seen from table 10·1, taken from Howard's report that 12·5 to 17 per cent of the entire weight of two samples of partly dried fish after 2 to 3 days in the sun was made up of the weight of the fly larvae in it.

It was estimated that at the time this survey was made the amount of fish caught in the Chad area and available for export to other parts of Africa where the protein it contained was urgently needed

10·2 Ostrich biltong drying indoors. Drying
of flesh by long exposure to the air produces
a 'leathery' texture and may also
lead to infection.

was about 20,000 tons and was worth about £2,500,000 a year. Yet
simply because the facilities of food technology were not available
to process it, a major part was lost and never reached the consumers
for whom it was intended.

The scientific principles used in all food technology are basically
simple. The main reason why foods deteriorate when they are kept
is because, just as they serve for the nutrition of man, so too are
they suited to the support and growth of insects and micro-
organisms. Perhaps the most ancient method of making them un-
available to such living entities is to remove so much water from
them, either directly or indirectly, that insufficient remains to
support the life of either an insect or a micro-organism.

All living cells on earth require moisture for their metabolism.
Cereal grains when brought in from the field, although they may
appear to be dry, may contain 20 per cent of moisture or more. If
they are stored in a bin thus, there is sufficient moisture in them to
support several varieties of insects. These insects will, therefore,
live and breed and, as they grow and eat the grain, it provides them
with biological energy for their life processes. This energy will, just
as in man, become manifest as heat. Since the bulk of the grain acts
as an insulator, the temperature surrounding the colony of insects
will rise so that, not only is part of the grain spoiled by the direct
attack of the insects but more may be damaged by the heat.
Sometimes, the temperature may even rise to the point where the
stored grain catches fire. For safe storage, grain must be dried until
its moisture content is 13 per cent or less.

Traditional arts of food preservation took advantage of this
principle in a number of ways. The plant seeds, wheat, rye, rice,
barley, millet, maize, are themselves structures evolved by nature
to provide stored food. The starch of their endosperm is used
for the nourishment of the embryo during the time it over-winters
(if it is a plant of the Temperate Zone) and until its new leaves
have grown and their chlorophyll can trap energy from the
sunlight to nourish the new-grown plant. The separation by
thrashing and winnowing is, therefore, to some degree part of a

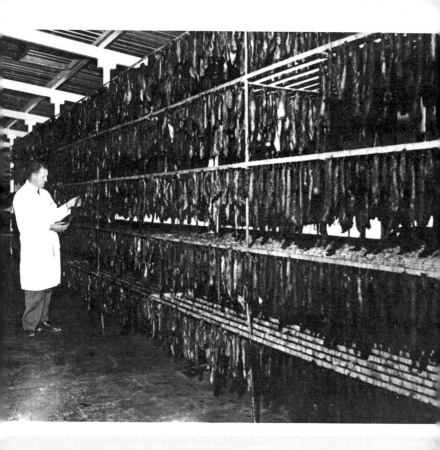

Table 10·1 Examination of two typical partly sun-dried *Giwan ruwa* (*Lates niloticus*) at Baga after 2–3 days' drying

Sample	Weight of partially dried fish (g)	Approximate number of fly larvae inside fish	Approximate weight of larvae (g)
A	1,130	1,954	140
B	1,760	2,523	226

technique of food preservation.

The direct drying of other foods has also been used. Fish has been dried in many parts of the world besides Africa. Slices of dried meat are prepared by numerous races. Biltong, a form of dried meat, was a customary food for travellers. The drying of meat or fish, either in the sun or over a fire, quite apart from the degree to which it exposes the food to infection by bacteria and infestation by insects, tends also to harm its quality. As was described in chapter 2, proteins are complex molecular structures which are readily disrupted. This is the reason why dried meat becomes tough and can, with some scientific justification, be likened to leather.

The principle of *osmosis* decrees that when two solutions are separated by a semi-permeable membrane and when one solution contains a higher molecular concentration of dissolved substances than the other, water will pass through the membrane from the more dilute into the more concentrated solution. For example, if salt is sprinkled on to a block of pressed baker's yeast, the liquid plasma which fills the living yeast cells will contain a lower concentration of dissolved ions than the damp salt outside and the liquid contents of the cells will be drawn through the semi-permeable membrane which forms the outer 'skin' of the cells with the result that the block of yeast, previously made up of a firm mass of cells, each with its own integrity and like a pile of grapes on a microscopic scale, is immediately liquefied. In consequence, the yeast cells, deprived of their moisture – that is to say 'dried' – die. Salting, which has been employed as a traditional means of preserving a wide variety of foods, from fish of various sorts to green beans, can therefore be considered to be an indirect means of drying. The foods are not in fact dried, nevertheless the water they contain is, in effect, withdrawn from their cells. Furthermore, the high concentration of salt constitutes an environment in which microorganisms which would otherwise cause decay are unable to subsist because they also are 'dried'. The preservation of fruit by boiling them in concentrated sugar solution, as is done in making jam, is another example of the same principle.

10·3 Osmosis is a process by which water can be 'sucked' out of the cells of an organism.

175

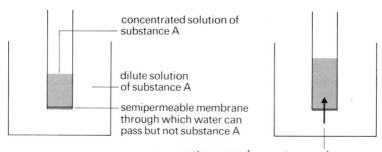

concentrated solution of substance A

dilute solution of substance A

semipermeable membrane through which water can pass but not substance A

water passes from outer vessel through membrane into inner vessel

The technical process of drying foods indirectly by pickling them in the strong salt solutions commonly called 'brine' does less harm to the protein than straightforward drying, particularly if this is carried out at high temperatures. It is for this reason that many of the typical drying processes are not taken to completion. That is to say, the outer parts may be dried leaving a moist inner section. Under these circumstances, preservation is only partial. The dried food keeps longer than it would have undried but it cannot be kept indefinitely. For this reason, traditional processes are to be found in many parts of the world in which a combination of partial drying and pickling in brine is used. Quite often the drying involves exposure to smoke. Foods treated in this way are, besides fish of various sorts, bacon, hams and numerous types of sausages.

Such traditional methods of food technology have performed a valuable service in keeping foods from decay so that they can support those who eat them. Many such foods – smoked eels, salt pork, pickled herrings and the like – are also considered to be particularly palatable. There is some evidence, however, from modern scientific investigation, that these traditional food products, recalled by many people with nostalgic affection, may in fact contain toxic ingredients as a direct result of the primitive technological processes to which they have been exposed. For example in

10·4 'Cheddaring' of cheese. The curd is divided into cubes, which frees water trapped in the protein fibres, and dries out the cheese so that it becomes increasingly resistant to decay.

1964 a report appeared on the presence of the carcinogenic compound, 3, 4-benzopyrene, in smoked haddock and smoked salmon. Five to ten times as much of the same substance was found in meat boiled over a charcoal fire. Besides this toxic compound, the range of substances of similar chemical class found in these smoked foods was similar to that found in coal tar. 3, 4-benzopyrene has also been identified in smoked meat. The concentration at which it occurs, while significant, is nevertheless low and the direct relationship between smoked foods and cancer has not been demonstrated. The significant fact for a student of food science to bear in mind is, however, that traditional methods, even those that have showed their usefulness over long periods of time, need as careful reassessment by scientific study as do new techniques.

Cheese is a particularly interesting traditional process of food technology for preserving an inherently perishable article by dehydration. The coagulation of the 'curd' by increasing the acidity of the milk, brought about by the proliferation in it of lactic-acid-forming *lactobacilli*, although it changes the molecular configuration of the protein, does not produce so drastic a change as to spoil its digestibility. And the traditional processing, commonly called 'cheddaring', during which the curd, maintained at an appropriate temperature, is divided by knives into cubes, piled up into a mass and then re-divided, serves admirably to free the water molecules entrapped in the protein fibres and so reduce the moisture content to a level at which the cheese becomes a durable article, resistent to microbiological attack, and capable of storage times far beyond those of the milk from which it was made.

But here again, although cheese is an admirable food made by a process of great antiquity, there is nevertheless need for constant reconsideration of its chemical composition in the light of the advancing knowledge of food science and of the changing circumstances of life in the ever-advancing environment of modern industrialisation. For example, a widely accepted group of drugs used by doctors for the treatment of mental depression are the so-called 'mono-amine-oxidase inhibitors'. In 1959, C. M. Ogilvie pub-

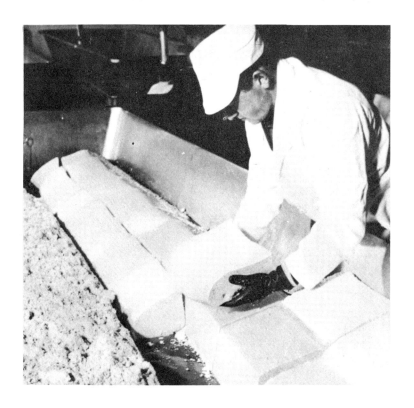

lished a paper in the *Quarterly Journal of Medicine* in which he reported that some of his patients who were being treated with these drugs were suddenly afflicted with attacks of severe headache accompanied by palpitations, flushes, sweats and raised blood-pressure. The cause of these alarming incidents remained unknown for eight years until, in 1963, it was discovered that they were always associated with the eating of cheese. The agent in cheese causing these violent toxic reactions was then identified as a particular naturally-occurring 'amine' called *tyramine*. It appears that under normal circumstances people have in their tissues an enzyme, an amine-oxidase, as it is called, which breaks down tyramine into harmless substances which are then excreted. Patients who are taking one of the 'mono-amine-oxidase inhibiting' drugs, however, are unable to carry out this particular process of biological detoxication and so suffer from the distressing symptoms which

10·5 The normal metabolic breakdown of tyramine. If the enzyme amine oxidase, which allows the first part of this process to happen, is blocked by a drug, tyramine is not broken down and has a toxic effect.

| tyramine | p-hydroxyphenyl-acetaldehyde | p-hydroxyphenylacetic acid |

I have described when they happen to eat a food with a potentially toxic amine, such as tyramine, in it.

An important point for the food technologist to bear in mind is that certain types of cheese are more toxic to these susceptible people than others. For example, Cheddar cheese is particularly dangerous. Certain Cheddar cheeses may, however, be eaten by patients on mono-amine-oxidase inhibitors with impunity. Others are immediately toxic. It has now been discovered that the concentration of tyramine in different batches of cheese from the same factory may contain widely different concentrations of tyramine. Values ranging from 0 to 953 micro-grams per gram have been observed. The reason for this, it has now been found, is that tyramine is formed in cheese during the course of the lactic acid fermentation which is an essential feature of the process of cheese-making. But the organisms, the *lactobacilli*, which are specifically introduced to produce the lactic acid, are not apparently those which produce tyramine. This, it seems, is due to one or other of the micro-organisms which gain entry by chance. Thus it now appears that this variation in the composition of cheese, a variation which may cause serious discomfort to a significant number of the people who may eat it, happens quite by chance and without the control of the manufacturers. In fact, unknown to the manufacturers, a substance of high pharmacological potential – tyramine – is being produced in fluctuating amounts.

Dehydration – that is to say, drying – is the main principle under-lying one branch of food technology; the use of low temperature is another. Just as the removal of water checks the activities of the micro-organisms causing decay, low temperature slows them down until, at freezing temperatures or thereabouts they are brought to a standstill. The use of low temperature to preserve food has been recognised since times of remote antiquity and historical accounts are to be found of ice being taken in the winter, stored, packed in sawdust or buried in pits, until the hot weather of the summer for use as a preservative for food. But it was only in the second and third decade of the present century that 'heat pumps' were invented which allowed refrigeration to be achieved by mechanical means. It is curious to reflect that the entire frozen-food industry and all the processes, such as the trade in large quantities of 'chilled' meat and the refrigerated storage of great quantities of foods of many sorts in ships and warehouses which depend on refrigeration, only became possible through the work of a retired captain of engineers in France who died of cholera in 1832 at the age of thirty-six. This was Nicolas Carnot who, almost unrecognised, made a fundamental scientific study of the nature of heat. The only work he published, *Réflexions sur la puissance motrice du feu et sur les machines propres à développer cette puissance*, which came out in 1824, was overlooked for a generation until Lord Kelvin drew attention in 1848 to its significance. It was, in fact, the basis of the theory of thermodynamics that made possible mechanical refrigeration in which an electric pump is used to compress a gas and then allows it to expand again.

A third main section of food technology involves the freeing of an article from the decay-producing micro-organisms which pervade the normal environment and then enclosing it in an impermeable container to prevent its being re-infected. The most generally used process is to get rid of the micro-organisms by killing them with heat and then protect the food thus sterilised by enclosing it in a sealed metal can. I propose to discuss these three processes, drying, freezing and canning, and their significance in further detail in chapter 11. Meanwhile there is a fourth arm of food technology that warrants attention. This is the use of 'additives', some to act as preservatives, which by their chemical action prevent micro-biological decay, others to prevent oxidation which produces rancidity or the interaction of proteins and sugars which gives rise to what is called the 'browning' reaction. Other additives prevent staling or delay the drying out of foods, others improve the structure and consistency of foods, enhance their flavour or serve as cosmetics to improve their appearance or colour. I have already referred to such additives as synthetic vitamins and amino acids designed to improve the nutritional value of foodstuffs and these will be discussed further in chapter 12.

In considering the battery of chemical additives which modern science has put at the disposal of food technologists and which are widely used in the articles which constitute the diet of the modern, crowded cities of industrialised nations, many people overlook the fact that only by making use of every advantage of technological ingenuity can a wholesome and attractive diet be made available to such great and populous centres as Paris, Tokyo, Manchester, Chicago and Moscow; they also overlook the attention and study devoted to the testing of additives for harmlessness and they over-look as well the toxic factors which exist – and which may be present in larger amounts – in foodstuffs deprived of such sophisticated agents.

Two chemical preservations which are generally accepted as safe by the public health authorities in most advanced countries are sulphur dioxide and benzoic acid. Sulphur dioxide is commonly permitted in sausages, minced meat, fruit and fruit pulp, jam, gelatin, wine and a number of other articles. There is little doubt that the general belief in its harmlessness to human health is justi-fied, on the basis of numerous tests. And while it is reasonable to prefer food fresh without any chemical preservative, it is interesting to note that, whereas of all the sources of food infection – so-called 'food poisoning' – meat products are the commonest, yet in Great Britain, sausages, in spite of their popularity and widespread distribution, come low in the list as foods responsible for food poisoning because of the use of sulphur dioxide in their manufacture.

The second most popular chemical preservative, benzoic acid, is highly effective in inhibiting the growth of yeasts and moulds in food. It is commonly added to concentrated soft drinks and is accepted without question up to a rate of 600 parts per million. It is also added to pickles and sauces among others of a long list of articles. Its general acceptability is not surprising. It has no taste or smell, it does its work well, and it has never been shown to have any toxic action on people. In tests on rats it has been added to their food in increasing quantity until 4 per cent of their total diet has been benzoic acid, yet the animals suffered no ill effect. But perhaps most consoling of all to those who feel doubt in using preservatives at all is the fact that benzoic acid is a natural ingredient of several foods and has been found up to a concentration of 500–1,000 parts per million in prunes and cranberries.

There are a number of other additives which are favoured by modern enlightened food technologists because, unlike purely artificial synthetic chemicals which in all prudence must be rigorously tested before being employed in food manufacture, they are natural components of unprocessed foods. Nisin, for example, is a modern discovery. It is a compound possessing antibiotic activity which is produced by *Streptococcus lactis*, an organism which occurs naturally in cheese. Nisin exerts a selective activity: it checks the growth of several organisms, for instance, certain *Staphylococci* and *Clostridia*, which spoil the quality of cheese, while allowing other organisms, which are useful in ripening the cheese, to grow. Besides being useful to cheese manufacturers, nisin is also added to foods that are to be canned because it is found that when this is done they can be sterilised without it being necessary to heat them to as high a temperature as would have been required without the nisin.

Another recently introduced additive, also accepted as being a harmless natural substance, is propionic acid. This compound prevents bread becoming sour and 'ropey' in hot weather. This defect is due to the growth of mould and of *Bacillus mesentericus*. Propionic acid checks the growth of these organisms. Its acceptance

10·6 Photomicrograph of a growth of the type of mould which often infects bread, especially in hot, damp weather.

was agreed with less doubt when it was found that it is a natural ingredient of certain Swiss cheeses – and it was observed to occur in human sweat as well.

Nevertheless, *a priori* arguments can never safely be applied to scientific matters and least of all to food science, a subject in which everybody's prejudices tend to run loose. It is just as foolish to reach preconceived conclusions about the safety of naturally occurring compounds (because they are 'natural') as it is to reach similarly unproved assumptions about the harmfulness of artificial compounds (because they are 'unnatural'). People accept certain foods and reject others for a variety of reasons. The fact that foods contribute to nutrition is only one reason; others are whether they are judged higher in desirability than clothes, houses, travel or any one of the thousand competing desires by which human behaviour is guided. Since the attractiveness of a food, quite apart from its freshness, freedom from infection and, last of all, its nutritional value, is an important consideration, we must accept that, in the current technological age, additives, used to make foods more palatable by contributing flavour, like saccharine, rendering them more attractive in appearance like the variety of synthetic colours approved by the list of diverse national public health authorities set out in table 10·2, improving their structure like the bromate and chlorine dioxide used in bread, and contributing to their nutritional value like the calciferol (vitamin D_2) added to infant food, the ascorbic acid (vitamin C) added to soft drinks, and the iodine added to table salt, are in need of careful study. And a main area of study must be the safety of such additives.

For any new chemical additive that may be proposed, it is now established practice to carry out a prolonged series of tests on several different species of animals. This type of biological assay involves at least two years' study, even when short-lived animals such as rats, mice or hamsters are used, and much laborious work by pathologists is done to examine all the tissues of the animals when they eventually die or are killed. Since there is no certainty that a substance harmful to one species of animal will affect another, even

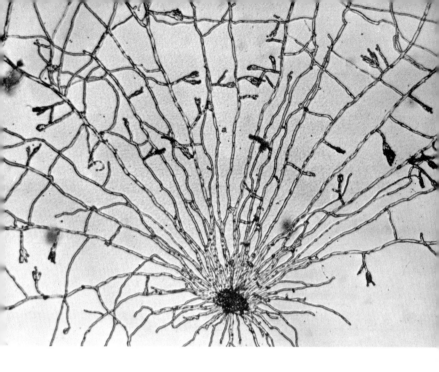

when toxic effects are found for the test animals, it does not necessarily follow that human beings would be affected, although it is prudent to assume that they would be. On the other hand, one could argue that even when a test substance has no effect on animals it may still harm people. In short, there is no such thing in human life as absolute safety.

During the course of the last two generations, food technology has advanced to a remarkable degree and the populations of many nations have benefited accordingly. Millions of cans of foods of diverse sorts have been distributed throughout the world and have provided wholesome and attractive nourishment. Frozen food, dehydrated food, foods such as eggs, meat and fruit transported under atmospheres of controlled gas composition, flour milled from scientifically selected grain to precise technological standards, fats from whales, peanuts and oil seeds, deodorised, hydrogenated, blended and manufactured into margarine, all these have served as a necessary part of the modern standard of living. In the achievement of so much that has been of advantage, it is not surprising

Table 10·2 Permitted food colours judged to be safe by the public health authorities in a number of different countries

	Great Britain	Australia	Canada	Denmark	Finland	West Germany	India	Norway	Spain	Sweden	Switzerland	South Africa	USA
Ponceau MX	+			+									
Ponceau 4R	+	+		+	+	+	+	+	+	+	+		
Carmoisine	+	+		+	+	+	+	+	+	+	+	+	
Amaranth	+	+	+	+	+	+	+	+	+	+	+	+	+
Red 10B	+			+									
Erythrosine BS	+	+	+	+	+	+*	+	+	+	+	+*	+	+
Red 2G	+			+							+		
Red 6B	+			+			+						
Fast red E	+	+		+	+		+	+	+	+			
Red FB	+	+					+						
Orange G	+			+								+	
Orange RN	+			+								+	
Oil yellow GG	+											+	
Tartrazine	+	+	+	+	+	+	+	+	+	+	+	+	+
Yellow 2G	+	+		+									
Sunset yellow FCF	+	+	+	+	+	+	+	+	+	+	+	+	+
Oil yellow XP	+		+										
Green S	+	+		+								+	
Indigo carmine	+	+	+	+	+	+	+	+	+	+	+	+	+
Violet BNP	+	+		+									
Brown FK	+	+		+									
Chocolate brown FB	+	+		+									
Chocolate brown HT	+	+		+									
Black PN	+	+		+	+	+	+	+			+	+	
Black 7984	+					+							

* For colouring whole, halved or stoned fruit only

that some few instances of error have occurred in this otherwise victorious progress of food technology. In 1932, Butter Yellow, a dye approved for use by the public health authorities of the United States, was shown to be a potential carcinogen. In 1946, it was found that 'agene' – that is, nitrogen trichloride – that had been used for a generation as a flour 'improver', produced in flour a substance, methionine sulploximine, toxic to dogs and several other animal species.

But these incidents cannot, of themselves, be used to condemn technological methods or to cast doubts on the competence of the methods used to test new chemical agents. Potatoes may contain up to 90 parts per million of the chemical compound solanine, of which 400 ppm has been shown to be poisonous. Onions have been shown to contain a substance capable of inducing anaemia; broad beans and horseradish are also potentially toxic, and there is a component of cabbage and certain other vegetables which tends to induce goitre. These are only a few of the 'natural' foods, which, judiciously used, can constitute an excellent diet. Nevertheless, the existence and properties of their less well-understood components need to be investigated just as do those of newly devised 'additives'. Rhubarb is an acceptable and agreeable article of diet, and yet, if it were only now being introduced from the Himalayas where it originated, no conscientious toxicologist would be prepared to approve of its use owing to the high concentration of oxalic acid in its leaves and stems.

11 Freezing, drying, canning and irradiation

Freezing

The technological development of freezing has been important for its own sake and equally important in making possible a new approach to food production in the technological environment of society in today's advanced industrialised communities. I have already referred to the historical significance of the invention of freezing machines dependent on the theoretical scientific discovery of what physicists call the 'Carnot cycle', in honour of its originator. This enables the food technologist to abstract heat from the commodities he wishes to freeze. The heat is taken out of these foods by three principal methods. 'Immersion freezing' requires the articles to be frozen to be plunged into a bath of some very cold liquid. At one time brine was widely employed, particularly for whole fish, but more recently other liquids have come into use, for example, solutions of invert sugar, which can be employed for freezing fruit. An alternative way of freezing by immersion is to put the food first into a metal container and then lower the container into the refrigerating medium.

A variation of this latter process is the use of so-called 'multiplate freezers'. These are in the form of a cabinet with a number of hollow shelves which form the freezing surfaces. The food to be frozen is put between the shelves which are then made to press upon it.

Perhaps of wider general utility is the method known as 'convection' freezing. In this process, the food is exposed to a violent blast of cold air which has been reduced to a very low temperature. Very quick freezing can be achieved by this means.

The technique of freezing is of itself a valuable method of preserving food for use. Refrigerating equipment not only allows the food to be frozen but also enables it to be stored at the most appropriate temperature for prolonged periods. Provided the freezing has been carried out under proper conditions, the quality and flavour of the frozen food when it is eventually used will be virtually indistinguishable from what it was when it was fresh. But freezing as a technique offers very much greater possibilities than merely those inherent in itself. Under modern industrial conditions, freezing requires the investment of substantial amounts of capital and the installation of large-scale equipment. To obtain a proper return from the capital investment, the freezing equipment, which is usually coupled with machines for wrapping and packing the frozen food, must be kept fully employed and to do this a constant supply of uniform material to be frozen must be available. Consider the effect of these various requirements on the manufacture of pre-packed frozen chickens. In order to insure operation on a large enough scale to guarantee an adequate economic return, the international financiers responsible for the operation need to set up, either under their own control or on a contract basis, hatcheries using eggs of a genetically standardised strain. The chicks from these hatcheries are raised in large-scale houses where they are fed on a diet compounded to provide the nutritional balance exactly suited to the growing birds and analysed to insure its proper energy value and its content of vitamins and minerals. The birds, reared on a predetermined schedule, are delivered at the appropriate time to the processing plant. There they are hung on a travelling rack, killed, bled, scalded, mechanically plucked, eviscerated, washed and chilled, packed in a plastic wrapper and then frozen. This whole process not only possesses the positive merit of efficiently, rapidly and hygienically preparing a valuable and attractive food product in a form in which it can safely be stored and distributed under controlled conditions but at the same time it possesses the negative advantage of signalising the end of what up till now we have called *agriculture*.

Up till now, food has been produced by one set of people, the farmers; sold to a second set, the merchants or wholesalers; passed on to a third, the retailer; purchased by the consumer by whom it has often had to be processed by being plucked, cleaned and decapitated. These are operations in which the purchaser not only has to do work on the article, it involves discarding a significant amount of the total weight which has been paid for. The modern

11·1 **Top left** Multiplate freezers with hollow shelves forming the freezing surfaces. The food, in this case, 'fish fingers', is put between the shelves which then press upon it. **Top right** Peas being individually frozen by convection freezing. The peas are frozen within minutes of passing the blast freeze funnel.
11·2 **Bottom** A poultry processing plant where everything, from plucking to wrapping and freezing, takes place as a single continuous operation.

innovation, derived from technology in general but owing much to freezing in particular, is the process by which a single organisation working, as does a manufacturer of motor cars, on an appropriate scale, is responsible for an entire streamlined process from the production of hatching eggs all the way to the distribution of processed, packed and standardised frozen chickens. This is no longer *agriculture*, it is *agribusiness*.

This transformation from agriculture to agribusiness is not solely dependent on the technological process of freezing. The same influences, that is, the need for a large supply of a standardised product capable of being processed in long runs by complex and highly automated industrial equipment, also apply to canning and the operations of dehydration. And should the preservation of food by radio-activity be developed into a practical and acceptable process, the same considerations will apply to it as well. But the revolution in which agriculture has been transformed into agribusiness is most clearly apparent. The systematised handling of chickens, from the genetical control of the eggs from which they come, through the range of operations during which they are grown up, killed, processed, wrapped and frozen, has reduced the cost and increased the supply of poultry meat until it has changed from a luxury article, only within the reach of those with money to spare, to almost the cheapest animal food. The effect of the same kinds of processes on peas has similarly converted them from an extravagant article available only during a short seasonal period, into a commonly available foodstuff on sale throughout the year. No longer is it necessary for a housewife to buy peas of variable quality, take them home and spend time in shelling them, which, besides the labour involved, compels her to discard three-quarters of the weight of what she bought in the first place.

Peas change in composition very quickly when they are growing in the field. In order to obtain the maximum yield and at the same time the best quality, not only must the appropriate seed be cultivated on land properly suited to its growth, but steps must be taken to assess the exact moment when the amount of sugar in the ripen-

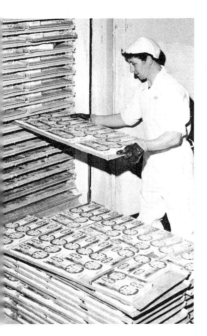

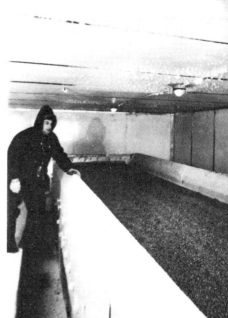

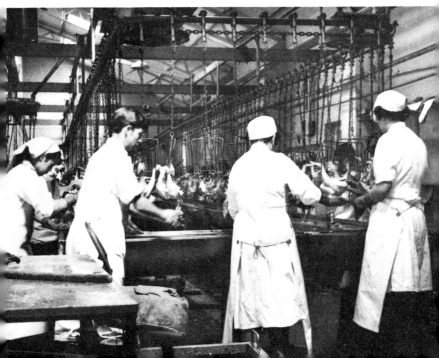

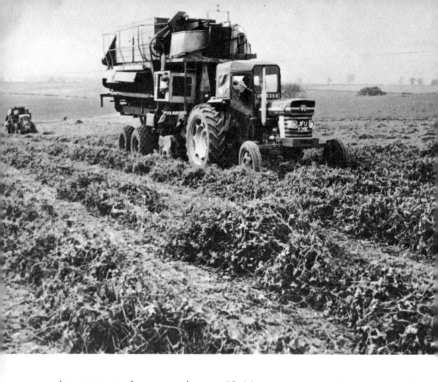

ing peas reaches a maximum. If this stage is missed, even by a day or two, the amount of sugar falls and the amount of starch rises proportionately. Under modern conditions, as the time for harvesting approaches, the peas are periodically tested by means of an instrument called a 'tenderometer'. Occasionally, sugar analyses may be carried out as well. At the moment when the optimum conditions have been reached, the whole crop is harvested mechanically, put through hulling and shelling machines and the peas are immediately frozen, usually on a belt freezer. Once they are frozen they can be stored for as long as necessary and packed in cartons as a systematic factory process without coming to harm.

The manufacture of 'fish fingers' is another example of the same principle. Of all foods, fish can, as has already been described, most easily go to waste when the processes of food technology are not brought to bear to preserve it. Besides its perishability and consequent uncertain quality, fish is troublesome to prepare and its preparation involves considerable wastage of heads, tails, bones and viscera. When proper facilities for freezing and processing are

11·3 Mobile harvesting of peas. The machines pick up and cut the vines, shell the peas and tip them into hoppers, all in one operation. Harvesting, shelling and freezing of peas must be done quickly at the exact moment when they are at their best.

191

available, the skinned fillets of such fish as cod or haddock are first packed in rectangular boxes in which they are frozen, usually in a pressure-plate freezer. The blocks of frozen material thus produced are then passed through a stainless-steel band-saw by which they are cut up, like pieces of wood in a sawmill, into 'sticks' $10 \times 2 \times 3$ cm. The frozen fish-sticks are then conveyed through a batter composed of egg, flour and skim milk powder, then through bread-crumbs, and are then passed through a continuous fryer. As they leave this part of the process they are immediately frozen again usually by being carried through a cold-air blast which reduces their temperature to $-40°C$ and holds them at this temperature for approximately one hour. Finally, they are packed in cartons in which, still frozen, they are distributed for use.

Here again we have a large-scale continuous process in which the functions previously carried out by a fisherman, who caught the fish and brought it to market on the quayside, by the merchant who bought the fish and transported it to a town, often some dis-tance away, by the fishmonger who bought it, and by the housewife who in turn bought it from him, cleaned and gutted it and then cooked it – all processes accompanied by greater or smaller losses – are now telescoped into a single, complex industrial operation. It is interesting to note that at least one large European firm manu-facturing fish fingers in this way nominated a director to the board of a major firm marketing furs. The reason for this is that in the systematised process which I have described the parts of the fish not used for human food, the so-called 'offal', are not wasted. The large scale on which the operations are carried out makes it economic to use these discarded parts of the fish for the feeding of mink which can profitably be raised in mink farms for their fur.

Drying

As I have already written, drying is one of the oldest processes used for the preservation of food. Before modern technological processes became available, however, it was an uncertain operation accom-

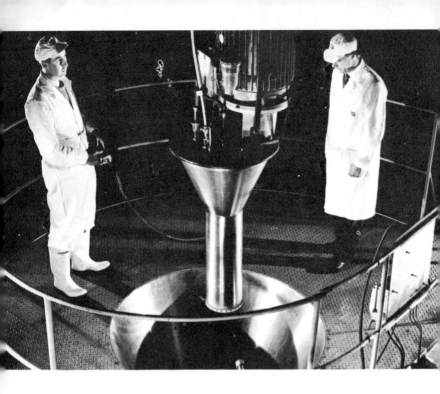

panied by capricious and often serious losses and usually involving deterioration in the nutritional value of the foodstuff concerned. The ancient and romantic process of haymaking, although concerned with the preparation of a dry animal feed capable of being stored from one season to the next is a good example of the scale of waste involved. To start with, the farmer making hay was dependent on the weather and on many occasions the weather failed him and his hay was spoiled. Before the days of technology, even if the weather was favourable the amount of labour involved in mowing the hay with scythes, turning it, piling it in cocks, opening the cocks, often several times to complete the drying, carting the hay to a barn or stack, building the stack and pulling it down again – all these operations involved an extravagant investment of human effort. Perhaps more significant than all this, however, was the need to grow the hay to an advanced stage of ripeness, during which its feeding value in terms of starch equivalent, protein and vitamin-A

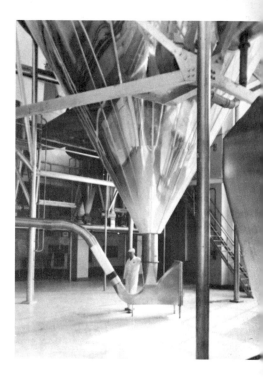

11·4 Spray-drying milk.
Left An atomiser spraying skim milk into a chamber.
Right Hot air is blown up from the lower end of the chamber, where the falling drops are dried almost instantly and are continuously removed from the bottom in the form of powder.

activity fell to a fraction of their maximum values, representing a major loss in effective yield per hectare of land.

The advent of the forced-draft drier, the tractor and its pick-up equipment and of scientific knowledge have in modern times permitted the manufacture of feed yields several times greater in terms of dried grass. The same material increases in the production of human food have been achieved by the application of the same principles. The commonest type of drying equipment for dehydrating food is a chamber in which the food is placed on perforated trays through which air, heated to a preselected temperature suited to the material being dried, is blown by a system of fans. Numerous variations of this principle are also used to accommodate batch drying or to do drying of a continuous flow of material. For liquid foods such as milk, eggs or soup, heated rollers may be employed over which the material is allowed to flow; sometimes the heated rollers dip into a trough of the liquid foodstuff. Whichever method is used, the dried product is scraped off the rollers by a fixed knife and can then be packed as flakes or powder. A different technique by which milk, coffee and other liquids have been successfully reduced to a dehydrated state is the use of a spray drier.

In spray drying, the liquid being processed is injected as a fine spray, either through jets or sometimes by a rapidly revolving plate, in a chamber shaped as a cone with the large end at the top and the point at the bottom. Hot air is at the same time blown up from the lower end. The falling drops are almost instantly dried as they fall and are continuously removed from the bottom of the drier in the form of powder.

The techniques of drying are basically simple, the detailed technique needed to produce a dried product of high quality is, however, difficult and requires great skill and knowledge. For example, to produce good quality dried milk without loss of nutritional value and capable of quick and complete reconstitution, it has been found that if the liquid milk is first heated for a brief period to 107°C, antioxidants are generated in it which help to delay any development of rancid flavour in the dried powder. Similarly, the preparation of an acceptable dried potato powder which will quickly recombine with water when it is required for use was found to be by no means easy. One way of preparing a dried product of good flavour and consistency was found to be to peel and boil the potatoes and by this boiling destroy enzymes likely to produce undesirable chemical changes. The boiled potato is next passed through a machine similar in design to a domestic potato-masher. Then, by adding 0·05 per cent of calcium chloride to the mashed material, it could, it was found, be dehydrated successfully.

A remarkable example of the way in which what might at first sight appear to be a small technical innovation or trick introduced into a process already properly based on scientific principle may transform an indifferent or even unsuccessful product into an outstanding success is found in the drying of green peas. The traditional method of preparing a stable foodstuff from peas is to allow them to become fully ripe and then, after thrashing the harvested plants to separate the seeds, to allow them finally to dry in the air. This produces a food rich in protein but entirely lacking in vitamin C. Furthermore, the yield of food per hectare – like that of hay – is comparatively low. Attempts were therefore made to harvest the green peas and dehydrate them in a stream of air warmed to an appropriate controlled temperature.

The first attempts at producing dehydrated green peas were not fully successful. It was found possible by appropriate adjustment of the conditions of drying to preserve much of the vitamin C content and to obtain a palatable article. The main problem, however, was to produce dried peas which could be readily reconstituted with water when the time came for them to be cooked and eaten. The difficulty arose from the fact that, no matter how carefully the drying was done, the outer layers of the peas became dry first, and when they dried they formed an impervious skin through which it was found difficult both to withdraw the water from the inner parts during the drying process and to introduce water again when it was wished to reconstitute the peas and eat them. The problem was solved with what now, with hindsight, appears to be a simple and obvious idea. This was to make a hole in each pea through which moisture from its centre could pass.

The idea may be simple but its execution demanded considerable technological ingenuity. The peas had to be made to drop into indents in a plate, a multitude of needles, one for each pea, had to be inserted mechanically and withdrawn and the perforated peas then dried. On the basis of this simple idea, backed up it is true by close study of the biochemical phenomena involved, a product could be prepared capable of storage at room temperature in any suitable air-tight package or container, which, when reconstituted in boiling water, was practically indistinguishable from fresh green peas.

This basically simple yet technologically ingenious method of drying peas is a good example of a successful process; the resulting article is palatable and of good nutritional value. In addition, however, it is convenient to use and is, in terms of its food value and convenience as purchased, no more expensive than fresh peas. Indeed, since such dried peas can be produced in bulk and marketed all the year round, the technological process by which they are prepared provides a net increase in the effective amount of available food. An alternative process for drying food, though even more ingenious technologically and making use of somewhat more subtle scientific principles, has so far proved less successful in its purpose of bringing food within the reach of the society for which it is intended. I refer to 'accelerated freeze drying'.

Accelerated freeze drying is based on the principle that it is possible to cause the water molecules, of which the ice crystals in a frozen food are composed, to evaporate directly into gas without first being converted into the liquid state if when a frozen article is heated it is at the same time maintained in a vacuum. To bring about this process, the food is placed in a freeze-dryer which is a closed vessel in which moderately sized portions are placed on metal trays. The vessel is closed and the vacuum applied until the pressure drops to about 1 mm of mercury. A 'coolant' may be passed through the hollow spaces within the thickness of the plates in order to freeze the food, although raw meat, if it is subjected simultaneously to a slight squeezing action between the plates and if the vacuum is applied with sufficient vigour, will become frozen merely due to the loss of heat occasioned by the rapid evaporation of moisture.

Once the food has been frozen, the plates of the dryer pressing upon it are heated either by circulating hot water inside them or by means of an electrical element. This causes the ice to *sublime*, that is to say, it is converted directly into vapour under the conditions of high vacuum in the chamber of the freeze-dryer.

The operation of this process requires skill. Fruit and vegetables need to be scalded before being processed. The function of this so-called 'blanching' is to destroy enzymes which would otherwise cause deterioration. Vegetable foods which are merely to be deep-frozen are also often blanched beforehand. The proper balance of temperature and vacuum must also be maintained in freeze drying.

So far, only certain foods have been processed by this means, but the quality of many of these when reconstituted for consumption has been outstandingly good. Meat, some kinds of fish, particularly shrimps and prawns, chicken and certain fruits and vegetables have been freeze-dried to give products of excellent quality. There are, however, three drawbacks, two technical and one economic, which have so far prevented this method of preservation being adopted on a major scale.

The first problem arising in the handling of freeze-dried foods is that, when the moisture has been removed from their cells by the process of sublimation, the dessicated tissues, although their structure is unharmed, are extremely fragile. It is therefore, necessary to pack the dried articles in special containers capable of protecting them from physical damage. The problem facing the food technologist is, in fact, similar to that with which Egyptian undertakers were once faced in wrapping the embalmed bodies of the mummified dead. The second technical difficulty in handling freeze-dried foods also arises from their delicate cellular structure. This presents a large surface to the oxygen of the atmosphere. It follows, therefore, that there is a much increased propensity for lipids to react with oxygen with the consequent production of peroxides and similar compounds which give rise to rancid flavours. To avoid this reaction taking place, it is desirable to pack freeze-dried commodities in such a way as not only to protect them from mechanical injury but also to seal them from atmospheric oxygen. This is sometimes done by packing them in an atmosphere of nitrogen.

The third problem which, as I have now pointed out more than once, is of equal importance to a food technologist, as is the chemical composition of the articles with which he deals, is that the capital cost of freeze-drying equipment is comparatively high in relation to its throughput, and the running costs to produce the necessary vacuum, refrigeration, regulated heating and to control the entire operation are also high.

11·5 A canning factory. The empty cans are carried to the filling unit, where they are filled and sealed. The sealed cans are then sterilised by heat applied for the appropriate length of time. Canning is still one of the commonest ways of safely preserving and distributing food.

Canning

One of the most productive methods for the preservation of food has been canning. During the century or more since it was invented and particularly since Louis Pasteur in the second half of the nineteenth century laid the foundations of the science of micro-biology upon which modern canning technology is based, many millions of cans of a wide variety of foods have been successfully processed and safely distributed throughout the world to provide a non-perishable stock of foodstuffs. Canning has many significant virtues which have served well to improve the supply of food. For example, in general, only the edible part of the article to be pro-cessed is canned, and even when the bones, for example, of salmon are put into the pack, the processing conditions are such that they are rendered edible and, incidentally, contribute nutritionally valuable calcium to the diet of those who eat them. Secondly, canned food is stable. It can be stored for months without deteriora-ting and, unlike frozen food, it does not need to be stored in special stores and under special conditions.

This durability, which all the main technological methods of food processing – freezing, dehydrating, the use of radio-activity upon which research is in progress at the present time – are capable of achieving, has had a profound effect on the total production of food and on the economics of its production. For example, fish which was previously a perishable article saleable only within com-paratively short distances of the points at which it was landed is now an economic commodity which is bought and sold on the world markets and of which the price is dependent on the complex factors affecting international commerce. The major fishing nations of the world, Japan, the USSR, Norway and, to a lesser extent Great Britain, operate fleets of deep-water trawlers serviced by a large 'mother' factory-ship in which the fish caught by the trawlers can be processed, packed and frozen at sea, and when it is brought to land either marketed directly, stored and kept for a later season, or sent to markets almost anywhere in the world. This is only

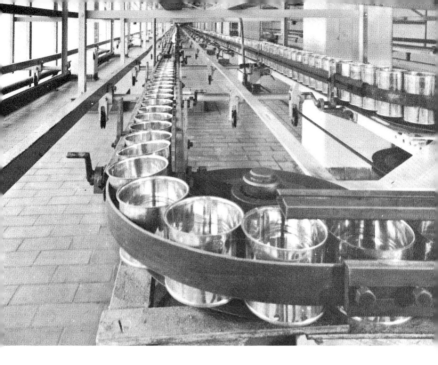

possible since the advent of modern technological methods. The same principle applies particularly to canned food. Canned meats, salmon and other fish, pineapple, fruit juices, a variety of food-stuffs some unknown before outside their areas of production, all have become available over a wide area. And this principle has a fundamental effect on the way in which food is produced for the market. Before the age of technology began, a man might set up a workshop to make carriages and could develop a successful business as a carriage builder. Today, no individual can hope to start a business making motor cars. Because of the high cost of the elaborate machine-tools needed to make such a complex machine, a motor car can only be manufactured successfully at an economic cost in very large establishments where cars can be mass-produced. This same principle is beginning to apply more and more extensively in the field of food technology. To manufacture tomato ketchup, canned baked beans or frozen 'fish fingers', equally large-scale plant is required. And to keep such plant fully occupied it is becoming increasingly common for the food manufacturer to control the growing of the tomatoes or beans, to check their quality and supervise their harvesting. The large producer of frozen fish nowadays will also own the fishing vessels which, equally with the processing equipment and the machines for packing cartons, are considered merely as one part of an integrated food manufacturing system.

An integral part of modern food technology is the way in which processed foods are packaged. Although in some respects packaging may be carried to excess and be used for unnecessary show or even to conceal the quantity of a particular packaged article, the general influence of modern packaging has been greatly to the advantage of the consumer. When Thomas Lipton, a small grocer in Glasgow, Scotland, started business in the middle of the nineteenth century, tea, sugar, flour, butter and most other commodities were dispensed from bulk supplies to each individual purchaser. The effect was that the food was often contaminated, the amounts dispensed were often inaccurate, substantial quantities were wasted and the amount of labour required to distribute each commodity was wastefully large. Lipton conceived the idea of pre-packaging his goods. Before long 'Lipton's tea' had acquired a widespread reputation and the original grocer's shop developed into a major commercial enterprise.

Within the same period of time, the distribution of milk, to name just one article, was also revolutionised; the fully automated pasteurisation and bottling plants have already been described. Complex machines for packaging sugar and flour, for the rapid and accurate filling of cans, or for wrapping bread, confectionery and diverse other articles are all essential parts of food processing. The recent development of so-called 'plastic' films has made it possible to protect semi-perishable foodstuffs such as bacon or portions of meat so that they too can be handled and distributed without wastage or contamination.

Although the basic principles upon which the practice of food technology depends are well established, progress continues at a rapid pace. For example, while at the present time plastic wrappers serve mainly to protect food from mechanical damage, from exposure to the atmosphere, from damp or from drying out, study is being made of the possibility of making plastic-wrapped articles more durable. The process of curing hams, for example, does not make the meat sterile although it very significantly reduces the population of micro-organisms which would otherwise accelerate deterioration. The practice is developing of wrapping hams aseptically in a plastic covering in order to protect them from recontamination. Thought is also being given to the possibility of adding an appropriate preservative or antibiotic. At the same time, research into the chemistry and technology of plastics themselves raises the possibility that in due course one may be developed capable of resisting heat. Such a plastic would not only provide a material from which hot-water pipes could be constructed – cold water can already be carried through buildings in plastic pipes – it would also allow food to be packed *and* sterilised in plastic containers and thus provide a light, strong and durable substitute for the sheet-steel can which has been used for packing food for more than a hundred years since canning was introduced.

Irradiation

I have already referred in passing to the use of radio-activity for sterilising foods. When this process was introduced it was hoped that it would enable articles of superior nutritional and dietetic quality to be produced since they would not need to be exposed to the relatively high temperatures required in canning to destroy decay-producing organisms in them. It would also have made it possible to 'can' food in plastic wrappers. So far, these hopes have not been realised. It is true that the ionising radiation emitted by radio-active isotopes, for example the gamma rays from cobalt 60, damage the reproductive abilities of insects, their eggs and larvae and destroy actively growing cells such as those in the sprouts of potatoes or the hearts of onions. Unfortunately, the use of radio-activity to sterilise foodstuffs has been found to possess certain disadvantages.

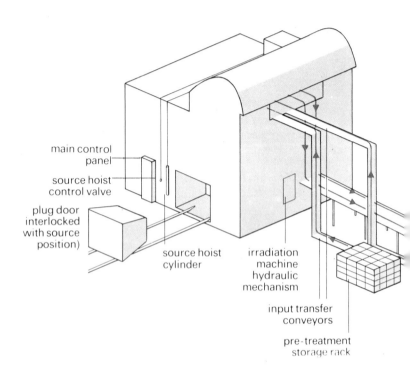

main control panel

source hoist control valve

plug door interlocked with source position)

source hoist cylinder

irradiation machine hydraulic mechanism

input transfer conveyors

pre-treatment storage rack

Although after exhaustive investigation it has been found that irradiated food is safe to eat*, if sufficient radiation is applied to sterilise it completely its flavour is so radically changed that people are not, under normal circumstances, prepared to eat it. For example, butter becomes bleached and tastes rancid and salmon loses its colour. Meat, on the other hand becomes darker in colour and its flavour is seriously affected; so much so that it has been described as possessing a 'wet dog' odour. If, however, foods are

* Recently a reassessment of the evidence has caused certain authorities to express doubts about the safety of irradiated foods.

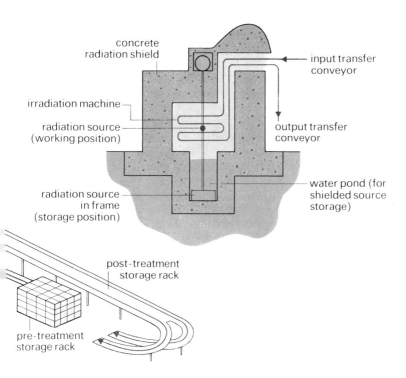

concrete radiation shield

input transfer conveyor

irradiation machine

radiation source (working position)

output transfer conveyor

radiation source in frame (storage position)

water pond (for shielded source storage)

post-treatment storage rack

pre-treatment storage rack

treated, not with 10 million rads of irradiation, that is, sufficient to achieve full sterility, but with only 3 to 5 million rads, most types of bacteria are killed. Even at this level (sometimes described as 'cold sterilisation') there is still some measure of deterioration in flavour and quality. This has been reduced by such steps as partial cooking of food before irradiation, or irradiation of food held in a frozen state while being treated. It seems, therefore, that ways may be found in due course to use 'cold sterilisation' without harming the food.

An even milder application of radiation has been used in an

attempt to achieve so-called 'radiation pasteurisation'. This has been done by irradiating to 1 million rads. This is sufficient to kill *Salmonella*, the micro-organism causing food poisoning and, just as thermal pasteurisation renders milk safe and makes it keep better, so also does 'radiation pasteurisation' benefit the foods to which it is applied. Unfortunately, even when used at these low intensities, the treatment still has a tendency to produce 'irradiation flavour'. So far, therefore, although ionising irradiation has been used successfully to disinfest such commodities as grain or dried fruit being unloaded from ships, it has not been applied on any scale as a significant part of practical food technology.

The fact that a promising method, made possible by the development of the modern industry using nuclear energy has failed solely because of its effect on taste and smell may seem strange. After all, food is basically intended to nourish rather than to possess any particular gustatory character. Yet this is not really so strange after all. In developing countries, just as in prosperous, industrialised nations, people have very fixed ideas of what they like and what they consider acceptable. A significant proportion of the total effort expended on food science is devoted to quality. One of the first mistakes made in the earlier years of the century when the principles of nutrition were being elucidated was to believe that people could be persuaded to eat what was known by scientific study to be of proper nutritional composition rather than what they accepted as constituting 'good' food. Whale meat introduced into Great Britain during World War II was refused by the population because of its taste in spite of the fact that its protein content is unexceptionable. Haricot beans, which were supplied as part of the protein provision in Vienna shortly after the war were, for the same reason, never fully accepted by the Viennese.

It is for this reason that food technologists have introduced diazo dyes as food colours, in spite of the need for rigorous testing to ensure their safety. Similarly, flour improvers, emulsifiers, synthetic flavours, egg substitute made from blood or fish protein for the manufacture of flour confectionery, meat tenderisers, preservatives

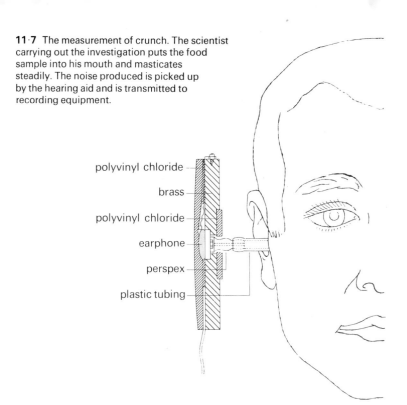

11·7 The measurement of crunch. The scientist carrying out the investigation puts the food sample into his mouth and masticates steadily. The noise produced is picked up by the hearing aid and is transmitted to recording equipment.

polyvinyl chloride

brass

polyvinyl chloride

earphone

perspex

plastic tubing

and humectants – all these have been developed to obtain consistency, flavour and colour, in fact, the 'quality' of manufactured food products.

Perhaps the most remarkable example of the application of advanced scientific study to food quality was some work carried out jointly in Sweden and the United States. Since one part of food quality is assessed by the sense of sight (its colour and appearance) another by the sense of touch (its temperature and consistency) quite apart from the judgment made through the senses of taste and smell, it is not surprising that attention has also been given to the noise made by certain foods when they are eaten, as apprehended through the sense of hearing. Toast, rusks, celery and potato crisps are all judged in part by the sound of the 'crunch' emitted when they are consumed. In work carried out partly in the Armed Forces Food and Containers Institute in Chicago in the United States and

11·8 The recording of crunch amplitude. The graphs show the different ways in which the amplitude of mastication sound diminishes.

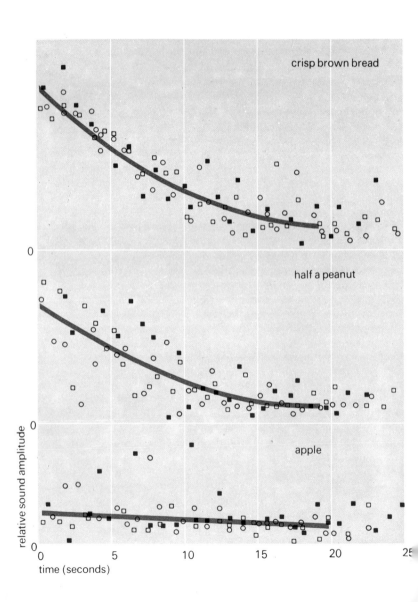

partly at the Swedish Institute for Food Preservation Research at Goteborg, Sweden, methods were elaborated to measure 'food crushing sounds' and standardise manufactured foods so that each produced the exact level of noise considered desirable. After a considerable amount of preliminary study, a technique was developed by which the gradually diminishing sound of different foods being masticated was recorded by means of an instrument similar to a transistorised hearing-aid which was, in fact, inserted in the ear of the experimenter engaged in chewing the different samples. This instrument was connected via an appropriate circuit to a magnetic tape and the record subsequently analysed for frequency and amplitude. By this means, standardised readings were obtained from such foods as crisp lettuce, bread of various sorts, beef, apples, peanuts, carrots, biscuits and wafers.

Figure 11·7 is a diagram of the recording device and figure 11·8 shows the curves obtained for bread submitted to various degrees of toasting.

12 Food synthesis and advanced techniques

Since the Second World War the British Ministry of Agriculture, Fisheries and Food has organised a survey of the different kinds of foodstuffs bought by working-class households. In the report for 1965, figures were given showing the rapid increase that was taking place in the relative proportion of so-called 'convenience' foods, that is, the products of the technological processes which have been described in the last chapter. Taking 1958 as the base line, the figures showed that the amount of frozen foods purchased increased by 147 per cent between 1958 and 1965. In the same seven years, the proportion of canned food and of food pre-packaged and processed, such as dehydrated soups and breakfast cereals increased by a sixth. And this trend is continuing.

But already there are to be seen new developments in processing methods. These are designed to render foods stable and capable of being stored and also to make operations such as plucking and cleaning chickens, peeling potatoes and removing the bones and offal from fish, previously done domestically, more efficient by carrying them out at a food factory. By so doing, it is often possible to make use of parts otherwise discarded and wasted. This trend is being taken still further. Platt, Eddy and Pellet have visualised the large hospital kitchen of the immediate future as a small food factory in which modern techniques such as quick freezing and accelerated freeze drying are used to conserve the nutritional value and palatability of prepared food or, indeed, of complete cooked meals until they are ready actually to be eaten. These can be stored until required and then prepared directly for consumption. Equipment has been designed by which a batch of frozen items taken from cold storage at a temperature of $-18°C$ can be heated to the serving temperature in a few seconds in a micro-wave oven.

These extensions of food technology designed to provide, not single prepared items like canned meat or frozen peas, each by itself, but instead prepared dishes or whole meals, represent developments of existing processes. The items are the same as those known before, only they are packed or otherwise processed to increase their stability, often to maintain a high nutritional value, and prevent the deterioration and loss which would otherwise occur. Some progress has, however, been made in developing entirely new foods.

The function of meat animals – sheep, cattle, pigs and the like – can be said to be to act as instruments to concentrate protein for the human diet. In scientific terms, however, the most efficient biological system for synthesising protein is the green leaf. Nowhere is protein synthesised more quickly than in a field of grass at its period of most rapid growth in warm wet weather. In terms of the recovery of nutrients from a unit area of land, it is grossly wasteful to allow the leaves of let us say, a wheat plant, to synthesise protein and other nutrients throughout the summer and then use only a minor fraction, the seed, and discard the rest of the plant. And even when the seed has been separated by threshing, a substantial part of it too is customarily wasted – at least it is not directly eaten by human beings – in the process of milling. If the cereal grain is not used as human food at all but is fed to livestock, the wastage of the total amount produced by the soil in the first place becomes larger still. In recent years a great deal of work has been done to develop a practicable means of using leaves directly as a source of protein.

The process requires the fresh leaves – many kinds may be used – to be passed through a pulper. The leaf juice is drained off and the pulp usually extracted once or twice more with water. The combined liquid is then heated to 70–80°C, which causes the leaf protein to coagulate. It can then be separated in a filter press. The dark green, cheese-like protein usually at this stage contains mixed with it 5–10 per cent of starch. It can be used directly as food, stored in a refrigerator or dried and ground, when it can be kept indefinitely if it is put into containers which protect it from atmospheric oxygen.

So far, although the technical process for manufacturing leaf protein has been worked out in detail and the nutritional value of the product established, the further development needed to convert it into a palatable and acceptable food has not been fully achieved. Work has, however, been done on a somewhat similar process,

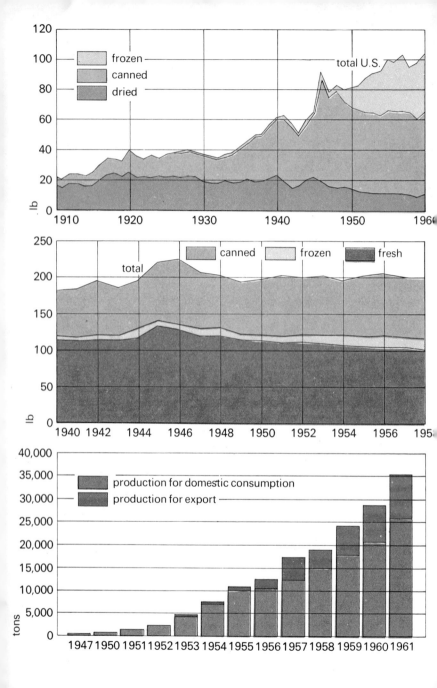

12·1 Left Processed fruit consumption (*top graph*) and vegetable consumption (*middle graph*) per person in the United States. The bottom graph shows the production of consumer packed frozen foods in Sweden.
12·2 Below The machine at Rothamsted, England, where leaves are processed, the juice extracted being used for the preparation of a protein concentrate. This is one way in which inedible material can be converted into nutritious food.

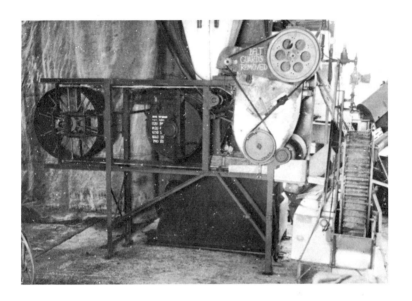

that produces from vegetable sources a 'spun protein'.

Two methods have been developed. In the first, filaments of casein, the protein from milk, or from soya beans or groundnuts, are prepared in an alkaline solution by forcing their dispersion through a fine spinnerette into a coagulating bath of acid and salt. The filaments are wound together into a 'tow', washed and treated with a binder of flour, gums and other ingredients. The bound 'tow' is then passed through a bath containing fat and flavouring materials and hardening agents to make it tougher or enzymes to make it tender. It is claimed that the result can be adjusted to simulate 'luncheon meat', steak or chicken at will.

In the second process, the protein suspension is extruded in the form of spaghetti and its consistency adjusted largely by means of the degree of heat to which it is exposed. Again, the final product has been made to simulate meat or various kinds of sausages.

12·3 Simplified flow-diagram of a process for producing algae. The plants grow in a liquid in the trough, which has a transparent cover to allow light to pass through. Carbon dioxide is brought in contact with the algal suspension in the gas-exchange tower and is then recirculated through the trough. Facilities are available for feeding in mineral nutrients and for harvesting a proportion of the algae.

A further attempt to short-circuit the use of animals in the production of attractive protein foods has been the elaboration of technical processes for the culture of algae for food. The principle behind this work is to obtain quick-growing plant substance all of which can be used for food without the need to discard stalks, roots, husks or other structures. It is also hoped to be able to grow algae with greater economy than normal food crops. The plant usually selected is *Chlorella*, which occurs in nature as the green scum on ponds and water ways. The principle used in Japan, Israel, the United States and Great Britain where work has been done on this project, is to cultivate *Chlorella* in a trough or pipe constructed from a translucent plastic material or covered in such a way that light can gain access. Carbon dioxide is introduced and the medium in which the plant is grown adjusted to contain the mixture of minerals required for optimum growth. Again, although some progress has been made, the process has not so far been brought to the point of a fully economic yield nor has the harvested algae been successfully converted into a palatable foodstuff. One special reason for food technologists to persevere in this research is the attraction which the process would have as a means of producing food in a space vehicle.

Yeast is a further possible source of protein to which food technologists have given some attention. The attraction of yeast as a source of food is that, although it requires a source of pre-formed energy to provide for its own growth, it can be propagated on sugar or some other carbohydrate which is frequently available in excess even in impoverished countries. If at the same time the yeast is provided with a source of inorganic nitrogen, for example, ammonia or ammonium salts – nitrogen not utilisable by higher animals – it will synthesise it into yeast substance of which protein is a component.

The commonest raw material used for the propagation of yeast, sometimes on a substantial scale, is molasses, a byproduct of sugar refining usually containing 50 per cent sugar. An alternative non-food raw material is the sulphite liquor residue from paper-making.

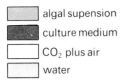

algal supension
culture medium
CO_2 plus air
water

gas exchange tower

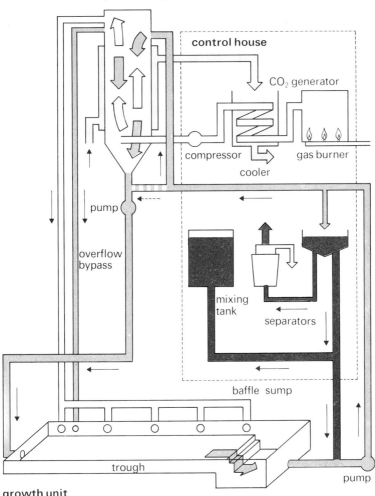

control house

CO_2 generator

compressor

cooler

gas burner

pump

overflow bypass

mixing tank

separators

baffle sump

trough

pump

growth unit

12·4 Photomicrograph of yeast growing on hydrocarbons, showing actively budding cells and oil droplets. The dried yeast contains 40% protein and can be used as an animal feed.

This contains sugars derived from the chemical breakdown of wood components. Before the yeast grown on this raw material can be used either as an ingredient of human food or for animal feeding it must be washed to free it from any possibly toxic contaminants.

An interesting recent development is the use of petroleum as a nutrient source for the growth of yeast. This provides a means of converting inedible raw materials, that is, petroleum and ammonia, into food or feed. This new process was made possible, first, by the isolation of a strain of yeast capable of utilising hydrocarbon, that is, petroleum or a particular fraction separated from crude oil. Two methods are, however, being used to grow the yeast for use. The first has been to culture the yeast on a particular fraction carefully selected from the main petroleum stream and then purified. This fraction is chosen specifically because the yeast can utilise it completely for growth. It follows, therefore, that the harvested yeast is free from residual or unconsumed petroleum. The purificent stage has, in fact, been carried out beforehand in the selection and separation of the feed stock.

In the second method for growing yeast on petroleum, a culture is selected capable of growing on a comparatively crude fraction. Consequently, the harvested crop of yeast is contaminated by unabsorbed petroleum residues or not completely metabolised substrate. Before it is acceptable it must, therefore, be purified by an appropriate extraction process or other means. By the use of these processes yeast can be grown on petroleum. The dried product contains about 40 per cent of protein and although it is unpalatable as a constituent of human food, it can take its place with such other materials as groundnut meal, fish meal and dried milk, as an ingredient of animal feeding stuffs. So far, no significant amount of yeast derived from petroleum has become available but pilot-plant runs suggest that it may be possible to produce protein by this means at a cost not significantly different from that of other protein concentrates used in livestock rations.

Although the use of otherwise inedible petroleum for the production of a feeding stuff represents a new development in food

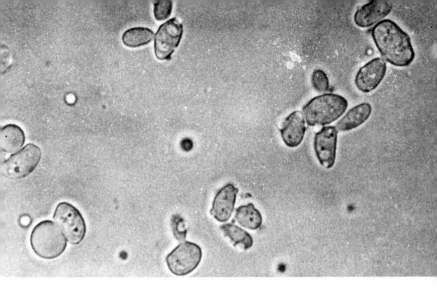

technology of significant promise for the future, a number of even more radical advances have appeared. These show that it is already possible to produce food by direct chemical synthesis and that this may become a significant source of food for future populations. During the first two or three decades of this century, great advances in nutritional knowledge occurred. Many new vitamins, for example, were discovered and the chemical structure of their molecules elucidated. In 1924, the American scientist Steenbock discovered that if the compound ergosterol, originally isolated in 1811, was irradiated with ultra-violet light it became converted into vitamin D, the rickets-preventing vitamin. But this early synthesis of a nutrient was merely a precursor of what was to come. In 1933, vitamin C, the anti-scurvy vitamin was brilliantly synthesised by Reichstein and by Hawarth and his collaborators. Riboflavin, part of the so-called 'vitamin B complex' was synthesised by Kuhn and Karrer in 1935. Progress continued rapidly. Vitamin A was synthesised in 1937 and in the same year nicotinic acid was recognised to be the pellagra-preventative vitamin and it was then recalled that this substance had been originally prepared as a pure substance in 1870. Vitamin B_6, also called pyridoxin, was synthesised in 1939.

Vitamins are biologically active components of food which, although essential for nutrition and indeed for the life of the consumer, are required in only comparatively small amounts. They are

also compounds of comparatively small molecular size. It is, therefore, not altogether surprising that, in view of their biochemical
interest and of their value as food components, the considerable
resources of organic chemistry deployed in their study led quite
quickly to their synthesis. Be that as it may, the manufacture of
synthetic vitamins has been of considerable value. A number of
industrialised countries including the United States and Great
Britain have public health regulations in force which insist on the
addition of synthetic B-vitamins to white flour. In less wealthy
countries, polished rice, which forms the staple diet of the main
proportion of the population, has been successfully enriched with
synthetic vitamin B_1. This has been done in the Philippines, in
Formosa and elsewhere in the Far East. Vitamin C is widely used
as an additive in soft drinks. Synthetic vitamin D is commonly
used as a supplement to dried milk preparations for infants. Synthetic vitamin A is added to 'Incaparina', a mixture of vegetable
protein foods designed as a milk-substitute to prevent malnutrition
among children in Central America. Synthetic vitamin A and synthetic vitamin D are added to margarine in most countries to bring
its nutritional value at least up to that of butter. And large quantities of these and other synthetic vitamins are used in medicine and
distributed as pharmacological preparations for the treatment of
deficiency diseases or the supplementation of diets thought to be
deficient in vitamin content. The large scale upon which vitamins
have been synthesised by the chemical industry has meant that the
price has continuously diminished. Under some circumstances,
therefore, synthetic vitamins must be accepted as an economically
rational means of providing part of a nation's food supply.

A further area in which synthetic chemistry, scaled up to a
manufacturing operation, is already in operation as a means of
supplying nutritional wants of large population groups is in the
synthesis of amino acids. The essential amino acid that is most
conspicuously lacking in many vegetable proteins is lysine. The
chemical molecule of lysine is non-symmetrical and it can, therefore, exist in two forms, as so-called *laevo*-lysine or as *dextro*-lysine.

In nature, lysine exists only as the laevo form. It follows that the lysine produced synthetically, which consists of equal parts of the two forms, is not nutritionally equivalent to lysine derived, for example, from meat. Research had, therefore, to be done to modify the method of synthesis so as to produce only the laevo form. This has now been achieved and the synthetic amino acid is available on a commercial scale. Experimental studies have shown that the nutritional value of wheat protein is significantly improved if it is supplemented with synthetic lysine. Diets made up predominantly of maize are improved when supplemented with both lysine and a second amino acid, also available by synthesis, tryptophan. The protein of rice diets is likewise made more complete by addition of lysine and a third amino acid, threonine.

The achievement of this further sophisticated development of food manufacture has already made a contribution both in human nutrition and in the preparation of feed for livestock, and the price of synthetic amino acids has been brought sufficiently low to permit their use in place of natural sources of protein of high nutritional value. Nevertheless, chemical synthesis requires considerable scientific expertise and access to advanced technological facilities. It is interesting to observe that the production of lysine, for example, or of some other amino acid in which a cereal-based diet is deficient, while it can be achieved by the application of chemical research, may also be possible by applying alternatively the science of biology.

Whether or not the chemical synthesis of lysine and other amino acids becomes a practicable process of food manufacture depends on whether it is found to be cheaper and easier to make them in a laboratory or a chemical factory or to grow them as food. Where a diet is deficient in a specific amino acid because it is largely based on a single vegetable food, for example, rice, maize or manioc, is it better to enrich this staple commodity with the missing amino acid? This is done in the Philippines for vitamins, when thiamine (vitamin B_1) is used to enrich the rice, and it is done in Great Britain, where it is added to the flour used to make white bread. Or is it a better procedure to educate the population to choose a more varied and nutritious diet and perhaps provide the poorer members with money to buy it? But, for the amino acid lysine, at least, there are several other possibilities. Although lysine synthesised by one or other of the methods to which I have already referred has been produced at a price sufficiently low to satisfy welfare authorities that it is worth purchasing, it is possible that these feats of chemical synthesis will be wasted. An alternative method by which lysine has also been produced on a commercial scale is by fermentation. This procedure involves the use of a micro-organism capable of synthesising lysine.

A second method, based this time on plant genetics, has been to breed a strain of maize – similar work is in progress with other cereals – the protein of which contains substantially more lysine than is present in that of normal varieties. This achievement was referred to in chapter 4.

But the whole question of whether or not the production of amino acids by synthesis is a method capable of making a major contribution to human welfare has changed, or at least is likely to change, following the work of S.W.Fox at the University of Florida. The starting point of this work were the studies of S.L. Miller in 1950. Miller was speculating about the origin of biological creation on earth. He prepared a mixture of the gases, methane, hydrogen, water-vapour and ammonia, which were probably present in the atmosphere before life existed, and he passed an electric discharge through the gas mixture. When he subsequently analysed the contents of the flask he found that small amounts of anything from eight to fourteen different amino acids had been produced. Miller took this as evidence of the way in which amino acids, which subsequently became linked together into protein, the basic component of the protoplasm of living organisms, had originally been produced from non-living components.

This piece of information remained for about a decade as nothing more than an interesting and thought-provoking item of circumstantial evidence. Then Fox and his colleagues, among others, took the matter further. They studied in detail the effect on this reaction of the exact conditions under which it was carried out. They investigated the effect of different temperatures and pressures and of the relative proportions in which the various ingredients were present. It was found that the fourteen amino acids which were simultaneously synthesised during the course of the reaction were exactly those found in nature in protein and no others. But perhaps more remarkable than this was the further observation that if this mixture of amino acids was subsequently heated to 170°C for about six hours, a light coloured polymer was produced which, if the conditions were appropriately adjusted, contained the amino acids linked in the same sort of way as they are linked in protein. This substance is now being called 'proteinoid' and the phenomenon by which it is produced 'pansynthesis'.

By the use of the normal methods of organic chemistry, the synthesis of protein presents formidable difficulties. Quite complex 'polypeptides' have been synthesised but these have always been far simpler in structure than natural protein. The simultaneous synthesis of fourteen amino acids, each one of which would require a series of closely controlled reactions of organic chemistry were it to be synthesised alone, and the subsequent synthesis therefrom in one reaction of 'proteinoid' granules, represents a very remarkable new development. 'Proteinoid' synthesised in this way has been found to possess many of the properties of natural protein. Its molecular weight is about 8,000, it is split up by enzymes which degrade protein and its component amino acids have been shown to possess nutritional value for rats.

Up till now, synthesis of such natural products as rubber or of products that simulate natural materials in the way that nylon or terylene simulate silk or cotton have required the molecules of each to be put together, if not atom by atom, at least in a systematic manner according to the intricate rules of chemistry. The possibilities arising from this new discovery of pansynthesis are, therefore, of remarkable interest and make the synthesis of protein something which may indeed come about in the future sooner than might have been imagined.

Now that pansynthesis has been discovered and its potentialities as a way of making artificial protein are being actively investigated, it is interesting to reflect on a rather similar process which as long ago as 1861 was described for the synthesis of carbohydrate. Because carbohydrate, although being the most important source of biological energy, is the commonest food constituent and consequently the cheapest of all nutrients, there has been little spur to incite organic chemists to develop a means of synthesising it on a commercial scale. Yet for more than a hundred years a potentially useful method has been known.

In 1886, A. Butlerow observed that when formaldehyde was treated with a mild alkali, a sugar-like substance made up of a mixture of components was produced. Since this so-called 'formose reaction' has been discovered, its mechanism has been studied in some detail. Much of this work was done by R. Meyer and L. Jäschke at the Technische Hochschule in Dresden. These workers found that when the appropriate conditions were maintained a mixture of the sugars, glucose, galactose, arabinose and xylose was produced. Fructose, one of the principal components of honey, has also been identified among the products of the 'formose reaction'. Although this process has not so far been developed to the stage of practical large-scale production, it does at least suggest that the synthesis of sugars and from them the further synthesis of dextrins and starches is a feasible target for research. Since formaldehyde, the starting raw material, is derived from natural gas or from coal, it appears technically possible – the economic feasibility is, perhaps, a different matter under normal circumstances – to envisage the manufacture of carbohydrate, as of protein and vitamins, from a non-biological source.

Fat, the third major component of food, is the only one to have been manufactured from non-food sources on a large scale. This was done in Germany during the 1940s when four large factories, one at Magdeburg, one at Witten, one at Heydebeck and one at Ludwigshafen-Oppau achieved by 1944 an annual output of 100 million kilograms of fat. The fat was made from coal. First of all the coal was submitted to the Fischer Tropfsch process. This was a means by which liquid fuel similar to petroleum was produced. A fraction boiling between 320° and 450°C – the so-called *Gatsch* fraction – was used as the basic material for fat production. Amounts of from 10 to 20 tons were put into cylindrical vessels, a solution of potassium permanganate was added as a catalyst and air was then blown in for a period of 24 hours while the temperature was maintained at 105°C. At the end of this time, about a third of the paraffins in the Gatsch oil had been converted to fatty acids.

The next stage in the process was to combine these fatty acids with glycerol in order to produce the esters of which, as was described in chapter 5, fats are composed. This operation was successfully brought about by heating the fatty acids in the presence of glycerol and of a zinc or tin catalyst. Considering the difficulties to be overcome, the synthesis of fat from coal achieved a remarkable degree of success. For example, the fat produced was refined so as to free it from any undesirable smell or taste of petroleum and, after having been refined, was converted into margarine. There were, however, two difficulties which in 1940 were not entirely solved although there is little doubt that in the light of modern chemistry, their solution could undoubtedly be reached. In natural fats, the fatty acids, although they may vary in the number of carbon atoms in their molecular structure from 4 in the butyric acid of butter up to 16 in the palmitic acid of mutton fat all contain an even number of carbon atoms. On the other hand, the fatty acids in synthetic fat are made up equally of molecules with even and odd numbers of carbon atoms. A more fundamental difference, however, is that 20 to 30 per cent of the synthetic fat is composed of fatty acid molecules which are branched chains, whereas in natural fats the molecular chains are unbranched. The synthetic fats were carefully tested on large numbers of rats, mice, guinea pigs, rabbits and dogs before being used as human food. Although there is no particular reason to believe that this difference in molecular configuration is likely to have any harmful effect, it is prudent to suspend judgment until the matter has been fully elucidated. Some differences in the

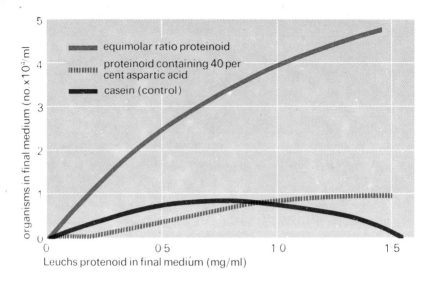

metabolism of the synthetic fat were, in fact, observed. For example, an increase in the amount of dicarboxylic acids normally excreted in the urine was noticed and among some of the people who ate margarine made from synthetic fat cases of nausea and diarrhoea were reported. Nevertheless, the point is clear that it is within the capacity of chemical science to make edible fat from such otherwise inedible raw material as coal and petroleum.

Protein, carbohydrate, fat and vitamins can all be synthesised and there is no technical reason why palatable foodstuffs should not be prepared from such synthetic nutrients. During recent years, the modern analytical technique of gas-liquid chromatography has been applied to natural flavours and aromas. It is true that it is not yet possible to specify in precise analytical terms all the chemical components which when combined together produce the aroma of fresh coffee, newly baked bread or Camembert cheese. At least it is understood that the tastes and smells of these commodities are exceedingly complicated mixtures. However, numerous organic chemicals have been identified as possessing at least the predominant characteristic of a number of different foods. These too can be synthesised and could be made available for combination with synthetic nutrients to allow technologists to manufacture if they wish a completely synthetic diet.

12·5 The nutritional value of synthetic proteinoids. The graphs show the growth of the protozoan *Tetrahymena pyroformis* on a medium of synthetic proteinoid containing an equimolar proportion of amino acids, when synthetic protenoid containing 40 per cent of aspartic acid was fed to the protozoa, and when casein (milk protein) was used.

What technologists are capable of doing and what they actually do may be two different things. Food manufacture is affected both by the laws of science and the rules of economics. There is an existing market for synthetic vitamins and for synthetic colours and flavours as well as for so-called 'improvers', anti-staling agents, humidifiers, preservatives, emulsifiers and the like. The large-scale manufacture of fats, proteins and carbohydrates is feasible and may well come about when they can compete – as synthetic rubber and synthetic fibres can – with natural biologically produced supplies. Certain American workers have already calculated the practicability of food synthesis as an extension of food technology. Their computation shows that to produce enough food to supply solely by chemical synthesis the entire food needs of 53 million people by which the world's population is at present increasing each year, an investment of 13,000 million dollars in chemical plant would be needed annually. Although this is seven times the current investment of the entire United States chemical industry, it is small in comparison with the sums spent on armaments or on efforts to fly to the moon.

While these figures indicate what is possible by the use of modern technological knowledge, what may well prove to be a more reliable reflection of how food technology may develop in the future is given by what has been happening now in the development of food supplies for the extreme conditions of space travel. Intense scientific study has been given to the problem and the solutions reached represent the ultimate in what can be done regardless of expense.

Perhaps the most direct approach has been to prepare a syrup containing the exact amounts of protein and fat, carbohydrate and minerals, and the concentrations of all the different vitamins necessary for the efficient functioning of the various systems of the body. This was in fact done as part of the Environmental Biology Programme of the US Office of Space Science. A cubic foot of this mixture was calculated to supply for a month 2,500 calories a day. This synthetic diet, however, has not been used in real earnest although it was tested over a full month by a group of volunteers at the Medical Sciences Research Faculty in California. The weakness of such a mixture, in spite of its carefully designed scientific composition, is that it is not attractive or even acceptable as 'real' food.

For astronauts engaged in actual flights as well as for the longer space journeys planned for the future, besides giving thought to the nutritional composition of the diet, the food technologists responsible for victualling space capsules also take into consideration the palatability of the items provided, their texture, whether they tend to break up into crumbs or otherwise deteriorate when handled and, finally, how best to package them. All these are factors which need to be studied by those dealing with normal problems. To provide for the specialised needs of space travel, however, the problems are all intensified. For example, for the quite prolonged series of orbits of the earth carried out by the American astronauts Schirra and Cooper, elaborate preparations including purees of beef and vegetables, or of peach or other fruit were provided. Similar commodities were also prepared in dehydrated form and were presented in wrapped bite-sized segments. Great attention was given to the composition of the wrapping material. Any food technologist marketing, say, biscuits (crackers) is anxious to avoid their breaking down into crumbs. Within the weightless environment of a space-capsule, crumbs are not only undesirable, they are downright dangerous since they might float about in the cabin. The wrappings for bite-sized portions of cheese sandwich and the like were therefore designed to be eaten and the plastic sheet in which they were wrapped was itself made of edible film so that the need to unwrap the pieces at all was avoided.

Ways of packaging the different constituents of meals or, if desired, whole meals themselves have been worked out. Where items are composed of dehydrated foods, a suitable water-pistol, designated as a 'pistol-type-probe water dispenser' can be inserted into the pack to rehydrate the dehydrated food. The work on the food technology of space travellers, while having to deal with the

Table 12·1 Proposed project Gemini menu

(a) Days 1–5–9–13

Meal A
Sugar frosted flakes
Sausage patties
Toast squares
Orange-
   grapefruit juice

Meal B
Tuna salad
Cheese
   sandwiches
Apricot pudding
Grape juice

Meal C
Beef pot roast
Carrots in cream
   sauce
Toasted bread
   cubes
Pineapple cubes
Tea

Meal D
Potato soup
Chicken bits
Toast squares
Apple sauce
Brownies
Grapefruit juice

(c) Days 3–7–11

Meal A
Strawberry cereal
   cubes
Bacon squares
Peanut butter
   sandwiches
Orange juice

Meal B
Corn chowder
Beef sandwiches
Potato salad
Gingerbread
   cubes
Cocoa

Meal C
Shrimp cocktail
Chicken and
   vegetables
Toast squares
Butterscotch
   pudding
Apple juice

Meal D
Beef with
   vegetables
Spaghetti and
   meat sauce
Toast squares
Fruit cake (date)
Tea

(b) Days 2–6–10–14

Meal A
All star cereal
Bacon and egg
   bits
Toasted bread
   cubes
Orange juice

Meal B
Beef and gravy
Green beans in
   cream sauce
Toasted bread
   cubes
Banana cubes
Tea

Meal C
Pea soup
Salmon salad
Potato chip cubes
Fruit cocktail
Grape juice

Meal D
Pineapple juice
Chicken
   sandwiches
Beef sandwiches
Chocolate
   pudding
Pound cake
   cubes

(d) Days 4–8–12

Meal A
Apricot cereal
   cubes
Ham and
   apple sauce
Cinnamon toast
Cocoa

Meal B
Beef bits
Potato salad
Fruit cake
   (pineapple)
Grape juice

Meal C
Orange-
   pineapple juice
Chicken salad
Peanut butter
   sandwiches
Peaches

Meal D
Mushroom soup
Chicken and
   gravy
Toast squares
Banana pudding
Apricot bits
Tea

peculiar problems of isolation, cramped space and the absence of gravity, can well lead to advances applicable to the problems of food technology for a normal environment. For example, such practical matters as the fact that tomato ketchup cannot be satisfactorily dehydrated, that the rehydration of prepared spaghetti may be hampered by a change in the chemical structure of the starch and that there are foods which cannot be successfully passed through the nozzle of a dispenser are all of practical interest.

A further circumstance arising from the technological investigation of space catering which may well prove of value in advancing food technology as a whole is the work that has necessarily had to be done on the food components which cause intestinal gas. It has been known by medical nutritionists that certain foods produce more flatus than others. Now, in studies particularly aimed at perfecting diets for astronauts, workers at the Western Regional Research Laboratory of the US Department of Agriculture have not only developed a method for measuring in quantitative terms the flatus-producing effect of different food components but they have also isolated a biologically active factor and gone some way towards identifying its chemical composition.

These are merely some of the respects in which the advanced technology being seriously developed for space travel is yielding results which, either directly or as 'spin off', are likely to be of service to food technologists and to the consumers who take advantage of their work. Other developments in this field are of boxes and containers which are themselves constructed of edible material and which, in consequence, save weight and space which would not otherwise be available for food. But regardless of the extent to which food synthesis and the various other novel and unusual procedures which have been developed by the scientific thinking of recent years come to be used in practice, it is clear that food technology as a whole plays a significant role in the provision of food for the nutritional wellbeing and health of the human community.

13 Food and health

The purpose of studying the composition and chemistry of the diverse commodities used as food, the selection of diets by different communities, the nature of nutritional science and the effects of nutritional deficiencies, and the achievements and successes of food technology – the reason behind all this effort is to bring health, in so far as it is affected by food. Yet health, even in its restricted context of nutritional wellbeing, is a concept that is not altogether easy to define. This is so even if we do not extend our search as far as Dr T.A.Lloyd Davies who, when he was professor of social medicine and public health at the University of Malaya in Singapore, wrote: 'if health includes freedom from pain and anguish then St John of the Cross was unhealthy. More than any other person St John understood the value of life. Health has little to do with freedom from hunger, pain or unhappiness so feared by man'.

This statement, nevertheless, has a good deal to do with the calorific value of flour milled to 85 per cent extraction rate and to the rent of houses for working-class families in Stockton-on-Tees. In 1755, Dr Johnson in his English dictionary wrote: 'health is the state of being hale, sound or whole, or freedom from sickness, pain or disease'. Or that it is 'welfare of mind, moral wellbeing, a state of salvation, purity, goodness or Divine Grace'. When allowance is made for its eighteenth-century turn of phrase, this is not altogether different from the definition of health proposed by the World Health Organisation in 1946 as being 'a state of complete physical, mental and social wellbeing and not merely the absence of disease or infirmity'.

The relation of nutrition to health can be considered at a number of levels. For example, a particular individual can be studied in detail in a metabolic laboratory. His calorie needs can be assessed by measuring his output of heat, either by direct or indirect calorimetry, and relating it to the energy value of his diet in relation to his body weight. The adequacy of his protein intake can be measured by recording his nitrogen balance while paying attention to the presently recognised needs for individual amino acids. In a similar way, the intake and excretion of an extensive list of vitamins and mineral nutrients can be studied and parallel analyses carried out on the concentration of these in his body tissues. But while the biochemical wellbeing of a volunteer undergoing detailed experimental study such as this can be guaranteed, the man or woman concerned can hardly be considered as living a full life even to the extent implied by the World Health Organisation in the phrase 'complete physical, mental and social wellbeing'.

At a second level, the nutritional status of a selected group of people can be studied. This is very commonly done by nutritionists and welfare workers whose business it is to investigate the adequacy of the diet of the population of a poor community, or of a special category of people living under some special set of circumstances. Nutritional surveys of this sort may be carried out by assessing the total quantity of the various types of food available. This may involve taking stock of the foodstuffs brought into the area and adding this to the tally of locally produced food supplies, making allowance for any changes in the amounts of stored food which may occur within the duration of the study. Alternatively, community studies can be based on an investigation of the amounts of food acquired by a sample of the different households of which the community is composed. Surveys may be made over some convenient unit period of time – a week is often selected. When the amount of food has been recorded it is converted into terms of nutrients by means of one or other of the published tables of food composition which are available for almost every type of food used in different parts of the world. Finally, the average nutritional requirements of the population surveyed are calculated, that is, the combined needs of the heavy workers, sedentary workers, adolescents and children together with those of the women of different ages, the expectant mothers and infants, for which assessments have been made by a number of groups of nutritional experts. Then, when the total of nutritional supply is compared with that of nutritional need, an estimate of any deficiency can be made so that the extent of any necessary improvement to the diet can be measured.

But although this is a useful way to assess nutritional adequacy

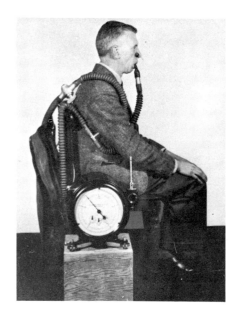

·13·1 Measuring the basic metabolic rate – the rate at which food is consumed by the body when no work is being done.

or to be made aware of nutritional deficiency, the method still provides knowledge which is limited in two main respects. First of all, the estimates of nutritional requirement drawn up by the Food and Agriculture Organisation of the United Nations, the US National Research Council, the British Medical Association and half a score of other authorities, while they are based on the best knowledge available, tend to be those amounts of the different nutrients known to be sufficient in the sense that for an average individual to take more would not do him any more good. That is to say, these scientific estimates of adequacy frequently contain a so-called 'margin of safety'. As I have written earlier, for a population to consume less of one or other of the dozen or so nutrients included in most of these tables may not justify including it among the list of that proportion of the world's population reputed to be 'starving' or even 'hungry'.

The further limitation in the value of surveys based on recommended allowances of nutrients when applied to mixed communities of people is that, even when the total amount of food available provides, according to the calculations of food composition, the average amounts of calories and nutrients recommended, there is

13·2 Heights and weights of school children in Glasgow, Scotland, between 1910 and 1959.

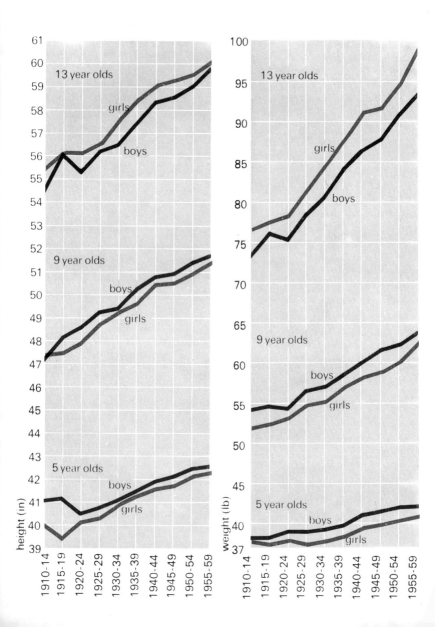

no insurance that the distribution of food to the individuals comprising the group provides each with a nourishing diet. For large communities, such, for example, as the population of India, or even that of New York, recommended allowances, though useful, may give a picture which is too favourable to one Indian (a poor workman, let us say, or a widowed mother) or to one New Yorker (perhaps a Puerto Rican, or a sick man out of a job) and underestimate the lavishness of the meals of another. The problem of insuring that vulnerable individuals within a family group or a larger community obtain their full needs is well recognised by nutritional workers.

There is another problem in food science that is frequently overlooked in considering the effect of diet on health. In the main, nutritional studies, whether they are carried out on individuals, families or whole populations, are restricted to some specific period of time. The third level to which study can usefully be extended is to the individual in the context of his lifetime. It is common knowledge that short periods of abstinence may do no harm to health and may indeed be of benefit. To miss an occasional meal cannot be called nutritional deficiency. The length of time during which shortage of one or other nutrient can continue without harm being caused varies. For example, considerable concentrations of the fat-soluble vitamins A, D and E may be stored in the liver so that deficiency symptoms will not occur until some months' shortage has elapsed. On the other hand, water-soluble vitamins can be stored to a very much more limited extent. So far as a total insufficiency of food is concerned, R. B. W. Ellis, studying messenger boys in Belgium during World War II, recorded that, although their growth and development was seriously checked by malnutrition during the war years, they quickly caught up with their contemporaries when adequate food became available in 1945 and 1946.

The difficulty of coming to a clear conclusion about the desirable composition of an ideal diet is underlined by recent studies on the growth of children. Every parent is anxious for his or her infant child not only to grow big but to grow big quickly. There is little doubt that a well-designed, or so-called 'balanced', diet, particularly one containing ample supplies of milk, allows children to grow and be healthy. There is some evidence, however, although this is by no means conclusive, that what is achieved by the most rapid growth is a shortening of the period of childhood and adolescence. One of the indications of physiological maturity is a change in bone structure. Professor McCance at 'Cambridge showed in 1953 that children given an ample diet rich in dairy products tended to be older in physiological age, as measured by X-ray examination of their bones, than was warranted by their chronological age. Some years before, Clive McKay at Cornell had found that rats given a properly 'balanced' diet but only in moderate amounts, grew somewhat slower but lived very much longer than litter-mates whose growth was hastened by more ample feeding. Whether or not these results can be applied to human beings, they at least suggest that the effect of diet on health deserves to be studied over the entire span of life. It would be a poor consolation for anyone to find that rapid growth during youth had to be paid for in a reduction in the span of life.

And this brings me to a matter in which it can most clearly be seen that, in spite of all our knowledge of food composition and of ways to process and preserve food, in spite also of our very considerable understanding of nutrition, there still remain areas of ignorance where our knowledge of the relation of food to health is lacking. Up till now, the food needs during senescence have hardly been studied seriously at all.

Man is an organism which is continuously evolving and which is at all times in a precariously balanced state of equilibrium with his environment. To maintain his equilibrium man is in a perpetual struggle – with micro-organisms, with his family, his workmates, his employer, with the other nations around him, and with the climate. Biochemically also, the cells of his body maintain an equilibrium with the nutrients of his diet. If a man does not get enough to eat, that is to say, if his intake of calories is insufficient, the normal 'basal metabolic rate' at which the life

13·3 The rate at which nine different physiological functions deteriorate with age. In drawing these graphs the efficiency at the age of 30 has been taken as 100 per cent.

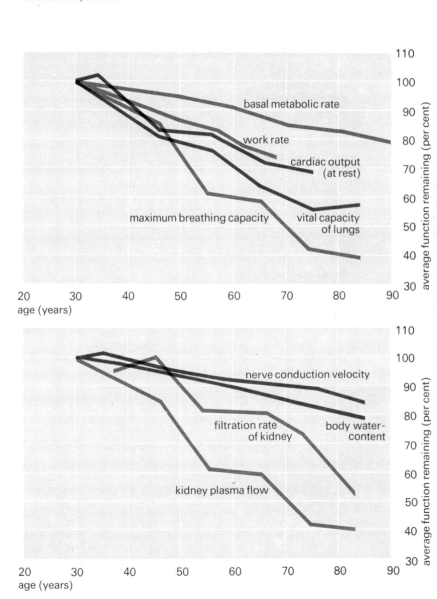

processes of his tissues 'tick over' will become reduced. This is an adjustment to reduced dietary intake. And it would be difficult for a nutritional scientist to say dogmatically that a man who had lost weight and then become stabilised at a lesser weight and a reduced basal metabolism was 'undernourished'. Indeed, he might even live longer under such circumstances. The problem becomes more difficult still when it is recalled that the equilibrium to which a man becomes adjusted is continually changing as his life progresses. The body dies a little every day. As time passes, the efficiency of the lungs, the heart and the kidneys continuously deteriorates, certainly from the age of 30 onwards and probably before. The elasticity of the skin can be seen to be less from one decade of life to the next. Brain cells die and are not replaced to an extent that 11 per cent of the weight of the brain is on average lost between the ages of 30 and 90. During this period, it has been reckoned that the number of taste buds in each papilla of the tongue falls from 245 to 88. This is one reason why people assert that no one can cook as well as their mother could when they were children. The bones also lose calcium and become brittle.

All these changes present a challenge to the food scientist. He is ignorant as to whether they are attributable in whole or in part to diet. He cannot say whether they ought to be accepted as inevitable or whether they represent a departure from 'health' and may, therefore, be preventable by dietary means.

The application of science and technology to the problems of human diets has achieved important results, particularly during the last two or three decades. Elucidation of the principles of nutrition has enabled public health authorities to make an end of the deficiency diseases of scurvy, beri-beri, rickets and pellagra. Great advances in agricultural science have enormously increased the productivity of farming. Some of these advances have been achieved by scientific research, by the breeding of new and more productive strains of crops, by the development of plant strains resistant to disease, by the production of higher yielding cows and quicker growing livestock. Other advances have come from the

synthesis of insecticides, fungicides and herbicides and by the for-
mulation of chemical fertilisers. A further step forward in the
productivity of the land has been due to technology: to advances
in agricultural engineering, to the designing of improved machines
of all sorts, to means of harvesting and drying crops, and to the
enormously increased productivity of the individual farm worker.
The parallel development of food technology which has been
touched on in chapters 10, 11 and 12 has further increased the
provision of food and at the same time improved its acceptability
and avoided the serious losses from decay and infestation which
take place where technology is not developed.

But in any consideration of science and technology and their
relationship to the health and wellbeing of populations, the most
important factor is, not the direct effect of science and technology
on food production and handling and the science of nutrition, but
rather the effect of technological thinking and practices on population numbers. The commonplace thinking about demography is
that scientific medicine and applied nutrition of themselves, by
reducing the death rate without directly affecting the birth rate, are
causing the world's population to increase and hence, it is argued,
numbers to outstrip food supplies with a consequent deterioration
in nutrition and health – primarily due, it is thus assumed, to the
very successes of science and technology. This is the so-called
'population explosion'.

There is no doubt that the various projections of the future
population of the world published by the United Nations Organisation and other authorities indicate that the numbers of people,
particularly in countries classified as 'developing', are likely to increase steeply during the next decade. In considering the relationship between population growth and the adequacy of the food
supply it is, however, important not only to study the effects of
chemistry and engineering on food production and on industrial
productivity and the whole way of life of communities as they
become increasingly affected by industrialisation. It is also important to reflect as well on the natural history of the human species.

236

Current thinking and the assumption that population increase must inevitably lead to food shortage is based on the *Essay on the Principle of Population as it affects the Future Improvement of Society*, which was published in London in 1798 and written by the Rev. Thomas Malthus. His idea, that human populations are restricted only by starvation, pestilence or war, has been tacitly accepted. The only addition to this list of checks on fecundity made by modern commentators is that of the contraceptive agencies recently developed also by scientific research. This simple approach to what is being taken as the main threat to nutritional wellbeing may, however, be an over-simplification.

There are many examples of human groups whose numbers are maintained in equilibrium with their environment by agencies quite other than starvation, disease, enemies or contraceptives. For example, in 1899, a German investigator, Kreiger, reported a study made in New Guinea of which he wrote: 'Though sterility is uncommon, and though the natives are fond of children, they raise not more than three, chiefly from fear of lack of nourishment, or because it is inconvenient or wearisome to raise them. Abortion as well as contraception is practised; and the fact that twins are scarce suggests resort to infanticide. It is abundantly clear that many primitive peoples thought in Malthusian terms long before Malthus. The women of primitive society knew all about Málthus's main point: that too rapid increase endangered support. Malthus's essay was essentially a learned inductive proof of an obvious thesis long understood and long acted upon'.

The situation existing in New Guinea was merely a single example of a general principle which, although it is often overlooked by modern nutritionists, applies today and applies to industrialised communities just as it did to the more primitive community studied by Kreiger in 1899. The idea that human populations are only restricted by pestilence, war or scientific contraceptives or, as the only other alternative, by famine does not make allowance either for the complexities of biological science or for anthropology. N.E. Himes, in his definitive monograph, *The Medical History of*

Contraception published in 1956, reviewed the diverse methods by which different races and communities in every continent have controlled their numbers. It is mistaken to imagine that merely because men and women have it in their power to increase their numbers in geometrical progression that they will do so until, like locusts, they eat up all the food on earth. C. M. Turnbull lived for a year among the pygmies in the rain forests of the Congo and described the highly sophisticated customs by means of which they maintain themselves admirably in balance with their environment.

These are non-industrialised societies unequipped with technological means of birth control but in which the population is kept stable by the complex interplay of human behaviour. There are equally numerous examples of so-called advanced communities – the Irish, the French, the British, indeed most of Europe and North America, in which biological fecundity is kept in balance by the equally valid group of ecological factors which together are described in the term, 'the cost of living'. This is a convenient omnibus expression covering the cost of space in which to live as well as the whole diversity of human needs, including food, upon which health and wellbeing depend. In one society it may include a 'bride price' or the trouble and expense of collecting personally the skin of a leopard. In another type of society it may include the price of a television set, an automobile or a house of the appropriate type to maintain the self-respect and social standing of the man or woman who acquires it.

There have been occasions, such as the present, when some major influence changes a previously stable equilibrium. The increase in living space brought about by the introduction of Europeans into North America initiated a period during which their numbers rapidly increased. The similar introduction of another animal species, rabbits, into Australia led to a similar result.

The establishment of the numbers at which a human population becomes stabilised, although it is influenced by the factors which affect animal populations as a whole, is also subject to peculiarly human forces. The nature of these forces is, perhaps, exemplified by

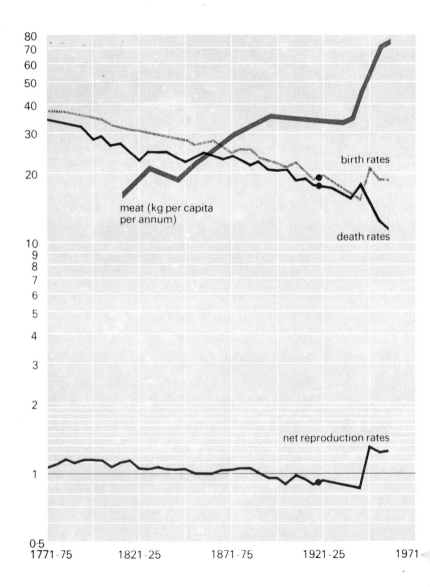

13·4 Average French annual birth rates per 1,000, death rates per 1,000, and net reproduction rates in the quinquennia between 1771–5 and 1956–60, compared with the annual consumption of meat and animal fat between 1812 and 1960.

an experimental situation which developed in Toronto, in Canada, and which was described by A. G. Huntsman in 1967. A mayor of the city bequeathed a substantial sum of money to the couples who could produce the largest number of children during successive ten-year periods following the bequest. Those who entered for these so-called 'stork derbies' bred freely to the maximum limit of human fertility. One winner was awarded a prize for a score of nine children in the measured decade. But after each race, when the ecological stimulus no longer operated and the prize was won or lost, the rate of increase returned to that current among equivalent populations influenced only by the normal social pressures.

These 'stork derbies' demonstrated in an extreme form the fact that human numbers are affected by wealth or the hope of wealth, among other influences, and the rate of increase may fall for complex social reasons quite apart from a shortage of food. It is often claimed that the rapid rise in population which occurred since 1945, and which it is also believed will lead to food shortage and malnutrition in Ceylon, was directly due to the technical efficiency of scientific public-health measures. The assumption, which has been made by a number of writers, was that the control of malaria which was effectively completed after the 1939–45 war was responsible in Ceylon for the dramatic reductions in the death rate and the sharp increase in the rate of population growth.

That the death rate from all causes did fall from 20·3 per 1,000 in 1946 to 14·3 in 1947 is true. But when the situation is examined more closely it can be seen that when the major reduction in death rate occurred, in the second half of 1946, less than one fifth of the population had been protected against malaria. And when the improvement between 1944 and 1947 is studied, it is found that mortality fell by 30 per cent in the malarious parts of Ceylon protected against malaria. But in those parts of the country naturally free from malaria and, in consequence, where spraying and other public health measures could have had no influence, the improvement in mortality figures was almost exactly as good, namely, 29 per cent. When Dr Harold Frederiksen looked into the matter even more carefully, he found that the death rate in Ceylon had been falling steadily long before World War II broke out. When a graph was drawn, it appeared that the dramatic fall of 1946–7 could be attributed much more reasonably to the increase in food imports and the consequent improvement in diet when the war ended than it could to the extermination of the mosquitoes which carried malaria. Indeed, over the longer term, the fall in mortality and the increase in population appeared to follow quite closely the nutritional quality of the diet. Food supplies had been increasing before the war; next, they fell while the war was in progress; and afterwards the improvement was resumed, coinciding with the abrupt improvement in health.

But Dr Frederiksen pursued the matter even further. He studied next the total economic activity of the population and observed that, not only had the prosperity of the people doubled, when measured in economic terms, between the years 1938 and 1951 when the mortality rate had been cut in half, but the parallelism between population and the wealth of the country was just as close as that between numbers and food supply. At the same time, the technical innovation of DDT spray to kill the malaria-bearing mosquitoes, far from being a crucial factor, seemed much more like an incidental attribute of the general change in prosperity.

Dr Thring, professor of engineering in the University of London, has for a number of years been concerned with the most advanced and sophisticated aspects of advancing technology, namely automation. For much of his work he is accustomed to drawing graphs of precise quantities that can be exactly measured. Lately, however, he has allowed himself a more speculative essay into the significance of the whole operation of science-based technology which is today being accepted by almost the whole world. In his latest graphs, Professor Thring attempts to relate the total amount of technology accepted by any particular community, a commodity that can be measured with some exactness, to the total happiness of the citizens, something which it is far more difficult to measure in units. Yet the measurement of happiness is, of all things, the most im-

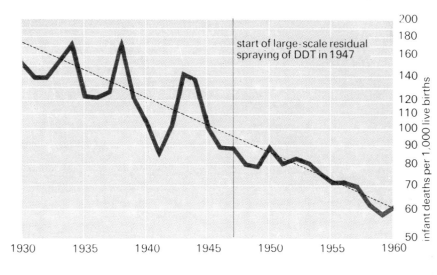

start of large-scale residual
spraying of DDT in 1947

infant deaths per 1,000 live births

200
180
160
140
120
110
100
90
80
70
60
50

1930   1935   1940   1945   1950   1955   1960

portant, since it is the purpose for which all the restless business of
the nation is done. At the bottom of the graph, when technology is
first introduced into a society, increasing amounts are accompanied by an increase in effective wealth and an increase in happiness. One aspect of happiness is an adequate supply of good food
and a correspondingly increased chance of children living out their
lives as healthy people rather than dying as infants or young adults.
But as the injection of technology continues to rise, the corresponding level of happiness reaches, first, a plateau and, later on,
begins to decrease. This fall in happiness occurs when the amount
of technology is such that the environment is contaminated by
fumes and noise, when roads are blocked with automobiles, the
skies filled with deafening jet aircraft, the countryside with mines,
factories, pylons and houses, and the food supply such that each
item is standardised and prepacked and the quantity available such
that the malnutrition of inadequacy is replaced with the malnutrition of surfeit and obesity. Ischaemic heart disease, diabetes and
varicose veins are a greater burden than rickets, scurvy, beri-beri
and kwashiorkor.

Frederiksen and a number of other workers have pointed out
that, although at the start of this curve, the increase in prosperity
and the improvement in health are accompanied by an increase in
population, this increase does not continue indefinitely. At the

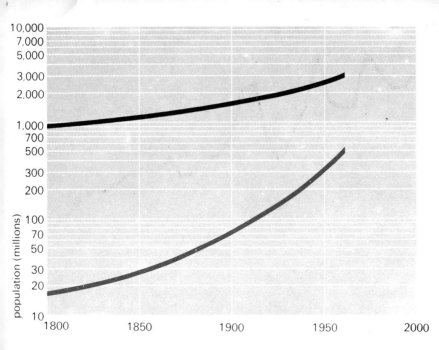

plateau, the increase slows down. Undoubtedly, the results of science and technology applied to the production of wealth and the preservation of health, as well as to the production and processing of food, have led to a large increase in world population. The crucial matter is the equilibrium numbers which will eventually emerge. For students of food science, this crucial question becomes: will there be enough to eat?

It is popular to assume – although serious thought is often lacking in making the assumption – that population increase must inevitably be halted by food shortage or even famine. We have already seen in chapter 8 that famines are caused, not solely by the lack of food, but by a combination of circumstances. It is equally true that there is little clear evidence that a high density of human numbers is accompanied by food shortage. Twenty-eight million people live in the 14,000 square miles of seaboard between Boston and Washington DC at a density of over 200 per square mile. Yet this is one of the most prosperous areas of America. In Hong Kong, more than 3 million people live on 389 square miles of territory.

13·6 The trend towards urbanisation. The upper curve shows the total population of the world between 1800 and 1960; the lower curve shows the number of people living in cities of 100,000 or more inhabitants.

243

And this is among the most prosperous parts of Asia. Holland, Belgium and Great Britain are crowded, and yet few of their people starve.

It is an over-simplification to imagine that each city or conurbation must provide its own food. In any social equilibrium there is a balance between agricultural production and all the other sorts of economic activity in which communities indulge. Although figures are not easy to obtain, largely because of the large amount of subsistence farming which still exists, there is a substantial body of figures which suggests that, whereas since the early 1950s the world's population has been increasing at a rate of 1·7 per cent, the enormously successful application of technology to food production – in the development of new strains of cereals, improved breeds of animals, irrigation, insecticides, fungicides and herbicides, and vastly more efficient machines – has at the same time increased food production each year by an average of 3 per cent. Even the United Nations, in spite of its preoccupation with the maldistribution of food, has accepted in the *World Economic Survey for 1967* that food production outpaces population. For example, the use in India of hybrid strains of wheat produced in Mexico has greatly increased yields, while high-yielding seeds, fertilisers and irrigation brought the Indian rice production from 46 million tons in 1966–7 to 62 million tons in 1967–8. And this is only a beginning. In chapter 12, I touched on a number of additional sources of food which so far have not been exploited economically; these include food synthesis from petroleum, the use of algae, the use of yeast and the use of leaf protein. In chapter 2, I referred to the exploitation of wild ungulates for meat and in chapter 4 to unused species of plants. Fish farming is a technology which is only beginning to be seriously considered.

If, then, the hypothesis be accepted that food shortage is unlikely to be the crucial limiting factor on population, it is important to consider what other circumstances are likely to come into play in the time ahead when the knowledge of food science, which has been the topic of this book, will come to be used. We can clearly see the beginnings of the restricting limitations which, although they may appear now to be little more than temporary inconveniences, may well grow up into major factors affecting the human situation. To a young couple in Boston, Paris, Tokyo, London or Leningrad, the difficulty in finding a house may appear to be merely one of the biological problems of growing up. To those who live and die in shanty towns on the outskirts of Lima or on the pavements of Calcutta, the reality of the 'population explosion' is more apparent.

One of the most consistent results of the application of scientific technology to human affairs has been the continuous growth of urbanisation. In every country to which technology has been introduced the number of towns with populations exceeding 100,000 people has grown and these have shown a tendency to coalesce into the great populated conurbations of the London area, greater Tokyo, the Paris region; even in empty Australia, the population, whose culture is firmly based on advanced technology, lives in the main in large cities. And it is in such crowded regions – in all, not one alone – and in every continent equally, that traffic – the problems of communication and transport – has grown into something more than an inconvenience. If the time comes when the circulation of large cities – the circulation of people, of goods, of sewage, heat, power and, most of all, of the products of the food industries – is strangled by their very size, the check on human numbers will not be due to food shortage but to a shortage of transport.

There have already been signs that this transport famine may be nearer than many people imagine and may arise from a lack of copper, an element present on earth in finite amounts. Copper is used to transport power and when temporary and local shortage has hampered the construction of power cables, the suggestion has been seriously put forward that silver, an element whose abundance on earth is even more limited than that of copper, might have to be used in its place.

The food scientist wants to do more than ensure the supply of sufficient food to provide a mere nutritional subsistence. His object is to ensure human excellence. Excellent human subjects cannot be produced without an abundance of cultural as well as material resources. Jean Mayer of the Department of Nutrition of Harvard University first summarised the facts from which it is reasonable to deduce that, of the shortages most likely first to restrict human development, copper comes before food. He also concluded that we are likely to run out of paper before we run out of copper. Since paper is an essential means of communication, without which it is hard to conceive the complex interlocked system of commerce, administration and government by which a modern technological society is maintained in operation, its lack could seriously curtail the development of civilisation. Furthermore, since to run an up-to-date nation requires a cadre of intensively educated people, a shortage of paper, without which such education could hardly proceed, would inflict further critical hardship.

My own prediction is, however, that the balanced biological system represented even by so complex and subtle an organisation as a modern technological community, modifies its development to meet its circumstances. When the death rate is high and the supply of capital and knowledge insufficient to provide mechanical power to assist a man's endeavours, he tends to produce a numerous family of children. When the death rate is reduced, and killing diseases mastered, knowledge and capital are amply sufficient to provide machines to do work and to provide amenities to make life agreeable, and when food supplies can be made available from every part of the world – as in France, the United States or Sweden – men and women do not produce families of sixteen or eighteen children.

If this prognostication is correct, how will food science develop in the future to satisfy the needs of the kind of society that can be expected within the next two generations? It is reasonable to assume that a significant proportion of the world's population will continue to live in a substantially self-supporting subsistence economy. Already, however, there is strong evidence to suggest that this proportion is dwindling and that, to an ever-increasing degree, the manufactured food products of world commerce will enter into the diet of even the most remote races. Flour, rice, sugar, dried and condensed milk, prepared fats, canned meat, fish and fish meal – these and other products of food technology are distributed to almost every corner of the earth. Furthermore, as I have already pointed out, the tendency of advancing technology is for a larger and larger proportion of the human race to move from the country-side and congregate in towns. And in such towns, in whatever part of the world they may be, the citizens expect to be able to obtain the same processed foods, the same canned meat and fish, the same products of the great processing plants which already distribute their goods world wide. It is my contention that this expectation is a reasonable one and will, in fact, be fulfilled.

Maryl Ballantyne, Consultant in Applied Nutrition to the Nutrition Division of the Department of National Health and Welfare in Ottawa, Canada, has pointed out that in the 1950s a large supermarket handled about 1,500 different types of food items. In the late 1960s, the number was 8,000 and by the 1970s it is expected to have risen to 12,000. Already, food manufacturers are seriously investigating the economics of using synthetic proteins and fats as ingredients; vitamins synthesised as fine chemicals are already employed. Margarine, in which fats from a variety of sources are processed to simulate butter, is widely distributed, and for the future the same principle will be applied to milk. 'Filled' milks, in which vegetable fats are substituted for the butter fat of the cream, are already manufactured; 'synthetic' milks, containing no milk ingredients at all are marketed on a small scale, so that their widespread use is entirely practicable if economic or technical advantage can be shown for their adoption.

The great fallacy in current thinking about food science is that there is one set of requirements for the technologically advanced nations of the world – where dehydrated and frozen peas, frozen chicken and canned pineapple are appropriate – and another for the less advanced 'developing' nations – where leaf protein, fish flour and 'surplus' dried skim milk are thought to be more fit. In fact, there are rich and poor people to be found in both developing and developed lands. The real challenge to the food scientist is to apply current understanding of food chemistry and nutrition so that articles of high quality, in every meaning of the term, are available to meet the needs of people no matter where they live in the complex, closely interlocked world of the present day.

Bibliography

2 Meat and Fish

Bacharach, A.L. and Rendle, T. (eds.) 1946. The Nation's Food, *Soc. Chem. Ind.*, London.

Borgström, G.A. 1962. *Fish as Food* (3 vols.), Academic Press, London and New York.

Fraser Darling, F. 1960. Wildlife Husbandry in Africa, *Scientific American* **202**, Nov.

Lawrie, R.A. 1966. *Meat science*, Pergamon Press, London, Oxford, and New York.

Maynard, L.A. 1946. The role and efficiency of animals in utilising feed to produce human food, *J. Nutrition* **32**, 345.

Pirie, N.W. 1967. Orthodox and unorthodox methods of meeting world food needs, *Scientific American* **216**, Feb.

Pyke, M. 1968 (2nd ed.). *Food science and technology*, Murray, London.

Simoons, F.J. 1961. *Eat not this flesh: food avoidances in the Old World*, University of Wisconsin Press, Madison.

Talbot, L.M. 1964. *Wild animals as sources of food* (Proc. 6th Int. Congr. Nutrition), Livingstone, Edinburgh.

3 Milk, cheese, butter and eggs

Folley, S.J. 1956. *The physiology and biochemistry of lactation*, Oliver and Boyd, Edinburgh and London.

Hawthorn, J. and Leitch, J.M. (eds.) 1962. *Recent advances in food science* (2nd Symposium on Food Science, Glasgow, 1960), **1**, p. 113, Butterworth, London.

Kon, S.K. 1959. *Milk and Milk Products in Human Nutrition*, F.A.O.

Rook, J.A.E. and Belch, C.C. 1959. *Proc. Nutr. Soc.* **18**, xxxiv.

4 Cereals, vegetables and fruits

Cruess, W.V. 1948 (4th ed.). *Commercial fruit and vegetable products; a textbook for student, investigator, and manufacturer*, McGraw-Hill, London and New York.

Kent-Jones, D.W. and Amos, A.J. 1957 (6th ed.). *Modern cereal chemistry*, London Food Trade Press.

McCance, R.A. and Widdowson, E.M. 1956. *Breads, white and brown: their place in thought and social history*, Pitman, London/Lippincott, Philadelphia.

Morris, T.N. 1951 (3rd ed.). *Principles of fruit preservation: jam making, canning and drying*, Chapman and Hall, London.
Pyke, M. 1952. *Townsman's Food*, Turnstile Press, London.

5 Oils and fats, sugars and spices

Deerr, N. 1921. *Cane Sugar*, Rodger, London.
McGinnis, R.A. (ed.) 1951. *Beet-sugar technology*, Chapman and Hall, London/Reinhold, New York.
Williams, K.A. (ed.) 1950 (3rd ed.). *Oils, fats and fatty foods: their practical examination*, (Bolton and Revis), Churchill, London/Blakiston, Philadelphia.
Winton, A.L. and K.B. 1932-9. *The structure and composition of foods* (4 vols.), Chapman and Hall, London/Wiley, New York.

6 The evolution of nutritional science

Davidson, L.S.P. and Passmore, R. 1963 (2nd ed.). *Human nutrition and dietetics*, Livingstone, Edinburgh.
McCollum, E.V. 1957. *A history of nutrition; the sequence of ideas in nutrition investigations*, Houghton Mifflin, Boston.
Nat. Acad. Sci.; Nat. Res. Council (Washington). 1953. *Recommended Dietary Allowances*, **302**.
Nutrition Foundation (New York). 1967. *Present Knowledge of Nutrition*, (3rd ed.).
Pyke, M. 1950. Industrial nutrition, Macdonald and Evans, London.

7 Deficiency diseases

Chick, H., *et al*. 1923. *Med. Res. Council*, Spec. Rep. Ser. No. 77 (London).
McCarrison, R. 1953. *Nutrition and health*, Faber and Faber, London.
Pyke, M. 1964. *Proc. 6th Int. Congr. Nutrition*, p. 54, Edinburgh.
Williams, C.D. 1933. *Arch. Dis. Children* **8**, 423.
Youmans, J.B. 1942. *Nutritional deficiencies: diagnosis and treatment*, Lippincott, Philadelphia.

8 Starvation

General State Printing Office, The Hague, 1948. *Malnutrition and Starvation in the Western Netherlands.*

250

Keys, A., Brozek, J., Henschel, A., Mickleson, O., and Taylor, H.L. 1950. *The biology of human starvation*, Oxford/University of Minnesota Press.

Medical Research Council, London, 1951. *Studies of Undernutrition, Wuppertal 1946-9*, Sp. Res. Ser. No 275. H.M.S.O., London.

Morgulis, S. 1923. *Fasting and undernutrition; a biological and sociological study of inanition*, Dutton, New York.

Woodham-Smith, C. 1962. *The great hunger; Ireland, 1845-1849*, Hamish Hamilton, London/Harper and Row, New York.

9 Social behaviour and economics

Asenjo, C.F. 1962. *Nutr. Rev.* **20**, 97.

Burgess, A. and Dean, R.F.A. (eds.) 1962. *Malnutrition and Food Habits* (report of an International and Interprofessional Conference, Cuernavaca, 1960), Tavistock Publications, London/Macmillan, New York.

Hames, P.J. and Robertson, E.C. 1954. *J. Amer. Diet. Ass.* **30**, 766.

Hathoway, M.L. and Foard, H. 1961. *Home Econ. Res. Dept.* U.S.D.A. No. **10**.

M'Gonigle, G.C.M. and Kirby, J. 1936. *Poverty and public health*, Gollancz, London.

Orr, J.B. 1936. *Food, health and income: report on a survey of adequacy of diet in relation to income*, Macmillan, London.

Pyke, M. 1950. *Industrial nutrition*, Macdonald and Evans, London.

Pyke, M. 1968. *Food and society*, Murray, London.

Rowntree, B.S. 1941. *Poverty and progress: a second social survey of York*, Longmans, London and New York.

Simoons, F.J. 1961. *Eat not this flesh: food avoidances in the Old World*, University of Wisconsin Press, Madison.

10 The evolution of technological processes

Asotoor, A.M., Levi, A.J., and Milne, M.D. 1963. *Lancet* **2**, 733.

Fraser, A.C., Sharath, M., and Hickman, J.R. 1962. *J. Sci. Food Ag.* **13**, 33.

Harslbarger, K.E. 1942. *J. Dairy Sci.* **25**, 169.

Kingsbury, J.M. 1964. *Poisonous plants of the United States and Canada*, Prentice-Hall, New York.

Pyke, M. 1968 (2nd ed.). *Food science and technology*, Murray, London.

Sebrell, H. 1930. *U.S. Pub. Health Rep.* **45**, 1175.

11 Freezing, drying, canning and irradiation

Drake, B.K. 1963. *J. Food Sci.* **28** (2), 233.
Drake, B.K. 1965. *J. Food Sci.* **30** (3), 556.
Hawthorn, J. and Leitch, J.M. (eds.) 1962-3. *Recent advances in food science* (2nd Symposium on Food Science, Glasgow, 1960), vols. 1-3, Butterworth, London.
Jacobs, M.B. (ed.) 1951 (2nd ed.). *The Chemistry and technology of food and food products*, **1-3**, Interscience, New York and London.
Pyke, M. 1968 (2nd ed.). *Food science and technology*, Murray, London.

12 Food synthesis and advanced techniques

Anson, M.S. and Poder, M. 1966. U.S.P. 2830902, B.P. 746, 859.
Bayer, R.A. 1966. B.D. 699, 692.
Conference on Nutrition in Space, University of S. Florida, 1964. NASA SP-70 (Washington).
Pirie, N.W. 1967. Orthodox and unorthodox methods of meeting world food needs, *Scientific American* **216**, Feb.
Pyke, M. 1968. Synthetic foods, *Sci. J.* 93 (May).

13 Food and health

Ballantyne, M. 1968. *Can. Nutr. Notes* **24**, 25.
Ellis, R.W.B. 1946. *Arch. Dis. Children* **21**, 181.
Frederiksen, H. 1960. *Pub. Health Rep.* Wash., **75**, 865.
Frederiksen, H. 1961. *Pub. Health Rep.* Wash., **76**, 659.
Frederiksen, H. 1966. *Pub. Health Rep.* Wash., **81**, 715.
McCance, R.A. 1953. *Lancet* **2**, 739.
McCay, C.M. *et al.* 1939. *J. Nutr.* **18**, 1.
Mayer, J. 1964. *J. Nutr.* Abs. **22**, 353.
Stone, A. and Heimes, N.D. 1956. *Practical birth control methods*, ch. 1, Allen and Unwin, London.
Turnbull, C.M. 1961. *The forest people*, Chatto and Windus, London/Simon and Schuster, New York.
Woytinsky, E.S. and W.S. 1953. *World population and production: trends and outlook*, Twentieth Century Fund, New York.

Acknowledgments

Acknowledgment is due to the following for the illustrations (the numbers refer to the page on which the illustration appears).

19 University College London, Department of Anatomy, photo A.J. Aldrich; 28 based on C. Merritt *et al* in *J. Agric. & Fd. Chem. 7*, 1959; 30-1 after F.Darling in *Scient. Am. 203* (*5*); 38, 202-3, based on M.Pyke in *Food Science and Technology*, John Murray, London; 47 Medical Research Council; 49 after W.E.Peterson in *Dairy Science*, Lippencott Co, New York; 51 Farmer & Stockbreeder; 54, 192-3 Milk Marketing Board; 55 (top) courtesy *Principles of Bacteriology and Immunity* by Wilson & Miles, Edward Arnold; 55 (bottom) R.J.Fullwood & Bland Ltd; 60 Zoological Society of London; 61 Poultry World, London; 67 Rank Hovis & Mc-Dougall; 71 National Institute of Agricultural Botany; 72, 74 after M.Pyke in *The Nations Food* (ed. A.L.Bacharach & T.Rendle), Society of Chemical Industry, London, 1946; 78 after A.L.Winton and K.B.Winton in *The structure and composition of foods*, vol. 1, John Wiley and Sons Inc, New York, 1932; 79 Government of Ceylon Information Department; 81, 105, 113, 114, 119, 120, 123, 125 Wellcome Museum of Medical Science; 85 (bottom) Tate & Lyle Refineries Ltd; 85 (top) British Sugar Corporation Ltd; 98 after G.H.Bell and J.N.Davidson *et al* in *Textbook of Physiology and Biochemistry*, Livingstone Ltd, Edinburgh; 99 Professor R.C.Garry, Institute of Physiology, University of Glasgow; 108 after L.J.Harris in *Vitamins in Theory and Practice*, University Press, Cambridge, 1955; 126, 164 Paul Popper Ltd; 133 Netherlands Embassy; 136 Mansell Collection; 139 Ministry of Agriculture, Plant Pathology Laboratory (by permission of the Controller of Her Majesty's Stationery Office); 141 cartoon by David Low, reproduced by permission of the Trustees & The Evening Standard; 132, 143, 144, 149, 153, 156, 229, 230 M. Pyke; 163 Radio Times Hulton Picture Library; 170 after T. Moran in *Nutr. Abstr. Rev. 29* (*1*), 1959; 173 South African Embassy; 177 United Dairies, London; 183 F.M.B.R.A.; 189 (top two), 190 Birds Eye; 189 (bottom) Fatstock Marketing Corporation; 199 H.J.Heinz & Co. Ltd; 205 based on B.K.Drake in *J. Food Science 30*, 1965; 206 after B.K.Drake in *J. Food Science 28* (*2*), 1963; 210 (top two graphs) Courtesy Economic Research Service. U.S. Dept. Agr.; 210 (bottom graph) after S.Martin in *Quick Frozen Foods 25* (*2*), 1962; 211 courtesy N.W.Pirie, Rothamsted Experimental Station; 213 based on G.Lusk in *The elements of the Science of Nutrition*, W.B.Saunders Co, Philadelphia and London, 1928; 215 British Petroleum Co. Ltd; 222 after M.Pyke in *Science*

Journal 4 (*5*), 1968; 233 after N.W.Shock in *Scient. Am. 206* (*1*), 1962; 238 after H.Frederiksen in *Publ. Health Report, Washington 81* (*8*), 1966; 241 sources from *Demographic Yearbooks of the United Nations;* 242 after K.Davis in *Scient. Am. 213* (*3*), 1965.

The graphs were drawn by John Messenger and the diagrams by Tamsyn Imson.

Index

Numerals in **bold** refer to illustrations